TEEN ANXIETY: DROP THE ROPE

*Evidence-Based Psychotherapy Guide
to break free from Tug-Of-War
with Anxiety*

Dr. Kinnari Birla-Bharucha

Dr. Kinnari Birla-Bharucha

ISBN: 979-8-9893582-4-3

DEDICATION

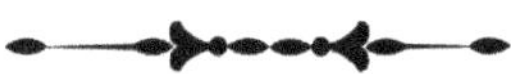

Friends, this book is for you - the villagers who raise our children. Moms, dads, grandparents, teachers, coaches, mentors - you shape our young ones with care and wisdom. Together, we build a community of guidance, empowering teens to thrive. Our shared duty is sacred.

To those who have waded through worry's tide and found shorelines of strength: Let this book be your lighthouse, beaming resilience through the dark. May its lessons steady you in struggle's grip and renew your spirit when strength ebbs low. Take heart, brave soul; the power to rewrite your story springs eternal.

Warriors who armor invisible burdens, this dedication is yours. Meet anxiety's gale head-on, for in the eye, calm abides. Each breath steadies your step through shadowed valleys into the light. Onward, valiant heart - the daybreak of joy awaits.

May you find the seeds of your own greatness!

ACKNOWLEDGMENT

Dear cherished readers,

Welcome to the transformative expedition through the pages of "Teen Anxiety: Drop The Rope." Life is a beautiful moment intricately woven together to guide us on a path of growth and evolution. Each person we encounter, be it a teacher, a validator, or a challenger, adds to our wisdom, skills, and virtues. I am deeply thankful to all who have been a part of my life and contributed to the creation of this book.

Let me begin by honoring the memory of my late father, Dr. Omprakash Birla. He was not just my dad but also my mentor, hero, and spiritual guide. His unwavering belief in me and his teachings of "love all, serve all" have shaped who I am today.

My mother, a formidable woman, taught me strength and compassion through her actions.

My husband, Vaikunth. His ambition and dedication inspire me to explore new horizons in my field. He is a role model of focus, determination, stability, security, and loyalty.

Let me introduce you to my guiding stars, Meera and Rayan. They have taught me invaluable lessons about time management, setting priorities, and finding balance in life. Motherhood, alongside my career, has been a beautiful journey of growth and love.

I am also grateful for my brother, who understands me like no one else, and my older sister, who has been an unwavering source of support as we adapted to life in the United States.

To my extended family, friends, colleagues, teachers, mentors, and well-wishers, I thank you all for your incredible contributions to my journey. Your support and belief in me have shaped my confidence and competence.

Special thanks go to my children's nanny and the staff at the school who have lovingly cared for my children. Raising them has been a collective effort, and I am grateful for the peace of mind they provide.

To my patients and well-wishers, thank you for allowing me to connect with you and learn from your experiences. Your presence has been a constant reminder to be humble and show up for others.

Lastly, I express my heartfelt appreciation to the team at Lincoln Writes for making this book a reality. Your editorial support, marketing efforts, and publishing expertise have been invaluable.

And above all, I am grateful for the divine's grace and blessings. To everyone involved in this project, your steadfast support has made this dream come true.

With gratitude and love,

Dr. Kinnari Birla-Bharucha

TABLE OF CONTENTS

ABOUT THE AUTHOR

Dr. Kinnari Birla-Bharucha is an esteemed clinical psychologist celebrated for her vast expertise and superlative impact on diverse populations facing a broad spectrum of emotional and behavioral challenges. With a doctoral degree from Adler University, she has dedicated her extensive postgraduate clinical practice to health psychology, emphasizing a holistic approach encompassing whole health and trauma-focused interventions.

Dr. Birla-Bharucha's professional journey encompasses both private practice and hospital settings, where she has consistently delivered comprehensive care to her clients. She firmly believes in integrating diversity, equity, and inclusion-informed factors into her treatment approach, recognizing the hearty influence of culture and social context on mental well-being.

As a first-generation Indian-Asian American woman, Dr. Birla-Bharucha possesses an elaborate understanding of the intricate nuances, unique challenges, and barriers faced by individuals from immigrant backgrounds. This firsthand knowledge fuels her passion for providing culturally sensitive and relevant care, ensuring that each person receives tailored support aligned with their needs.

Beyond her clinical work, Dr. Birla-Bharucha actively engages as a consultant and author, sharing her expertise and empowering others to transcend the limitations of a survivor's mentality. She fervently advocates personal growth and transformation, encouraging individuals to reclaim their agency and become architects of their own lives.

Drawing on over a decade of experience, Dr. Birla-Bharucha specializes in evidence-based therapeutic modalities, including cognitive-behavioral therapy (CBT), mindfulness-based practices, acceptance and commitment therapy (ACT), and inner child and shadow work. She seamlessly combines these approaches to provide her clients with a comprehensive healing and personal development toolkit.

Dr. Birla-Bharucha has made waves beyond her professional achievements. With a staunch commitment to her client's well-being, she creates a safe and non-judgmental space for exploration and growth. She empowers individuals to navigate challenges, discover their inherent strengths, and embrace a life of purpose and fulfillment through courage, resilience, and a deeper connection to their inner selves.

"Teen Anxiety: Drop The Rope" is a tribute to Dr. Kinnari Birla-Bharucha's exceptional expertise and dedication. In this book, she combines her vast clinical knowledge, compassionate approach, and diverse therapeutic techniques to provide a comprehensive guide for teenagers and their families. She offers invaluable insights and practical strategies to overcome anxiety and not just survive but live a life of resilience and well-being.

PREFACE

"My mission in life is not merely to survive, but to thrive; and to do so with passion, compassion, humor, and style."

- Dr. Maya Angelou

During my golden years of teenage life, where self-discovery intertwines with the intricacies of societal expectations, the pursuit of thriving can often feel like a far-fetched dream. During these formative years, anxiety can take root, casting shadows of doubt and uncertainty over the path to self-realization.

As a clinical psychologist and advocate for holistic well-being, I firmly believe that every teenager has the innate capacity to break loose from anxiety and bounce back stronger and wiser.

Only through passion, compassion, humor, and style can we unravel the secrets that entangle their minds, liberating them to reach for their true potential.

This book, "Teen Anxiety: Drop The Rope," invites adolescents, parents, and educators to embark on a transformative expedition towards a flavorful and empowered life.

Reflecting upon my years of experience and expertise, I aim to provide a comprehensive roadmap that combines evidence-based techniques, profound insights, and heartfelt guidance.

Within these pages, you will find a sanctuary of wisdom and practical tools to overcome the treacherous landscapes of anxiety.

From understanding the tricky workings of the teenage mind to exploring the powerful impact of self-compassion and mindfulness, each chapter is designed to empower teenagers and those who support them.

Together, we will break stereotypes, acknowledging that anxiety is not an enemy to be conquered but a messenger that beckons us to reclaim our power and rewrite our story. Through a blend of psychological expertise, personal anecdotes, and a genuine understanding of the teenage experience, this book aims to inspire and guide you toward a life where anxiety no longer defines but instead fuels growth and perseverance.

Remember, dear readers; you are not alone. Together, we shall help you drop the rope that winds so tightly around you, limiting you from reaching the epitome of your highest self.

CHAPTER 1:

INTRODUCTION

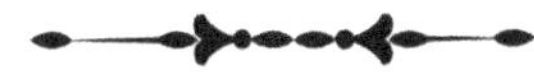

If you've picked up this book, chances are either you or someone you know is a teenager suffering from an anxiety disorder. I congratulate you as you've taken the first step toward recovery.

Did you know?

Based on National Comorbidity Survey Adolescent Supplement (NCS-A) findings, an estimated 31.9% of adolescents had an anxiety disorder. Of those adolescents diagnosed with an anxiety disorder, about 8.3% had a severe impairment that categorically affected their daily life. This prevalence was higher for females, with an incidence of 38%, than for males, which was 26.1%. Alarming.

Now, you might be wondering, what can be done to curb the damages done by this debilitating illness? Well, my mantra is:

"Our sorrows and wounds are healed only when we compassionately touch them."

My name is Dr. Kinnari Birla, a doctoral graduate of Adler University, and I have over a decade of experience as a clinical psychologist. I have attended the American Psychological Association (APA) accredited doctoral program for five years, defended a doctoral dissertation, and received over 4000 supervised clinical training hours and experiences in evidence-based modalities and psychological assessments. I have served patients with a varied range of emotional and behavioral disorders to a diverse population, all while maintaining cultural sensitivities. My expertise is in treating anxiety disorders, trauma, PTSD, moral injury, depression, bereavement, life transitions, self-esteem, dealing with low self-worth, chronic medical illnesses, and interpersonal relationship issues, only to name a few.

I take *Diversity, Equity, and Inclusion* very seriously. In therapy, I integrate scientific methods, evidence-based practices, and the art of psychotherapy to help you comprehend your illness and share therapeutic techniques to overcome them. I work from person-centric, mindfulness-based, cognitive behavioral therapy, interpersonal psychotherapy, humanistic/existential, and acceptance and commitment therapy modalities.

Allow me to be the catalyst in your life who provides skills and tools so you can practice psychological flexibility while facing life's adversities. In my vast years of clinical practice, I have experienced that the *power of connection* is the vehicle in the journey toward healing. I am a compassionate change agent who will assist you in recognizing your story, your challenges, your culture, and your path to acquire a better understanding of *you*.

With this book, I hope you will gain more insight into managing your challenges by understanding the relationship between your past wounds, present stressors, and future worries. By the end of this book, I promise we will find the strength within you so that you can live the best version of yourself.

My focus for this book will be Cognitive Behavioral Therapy (CBT) and Acceptance and Commitment Therapy (ACT). We will learn how you can use these treatment modalities to win the battle against anxiety.

Cognitive behavioral therapy, or CBT, stresses the role of thinking in how we feel and act. It revolves around believing that thoughts, rather than people or events, cause negative feelings. The therapist's job is to support the client in identifying, testing the reality of, and correcting dysfunctional beliefs underlying their thinking. In this way, the therapist helps the client modify those thoughts and the behaviors that stem from them. CBT is a structured collaboration between therapist and client and often calls for homework assignments. CBT has been clinically proven to aid clients with anxiety disorders in a relatively short period.

Acceptance and Commitment Therapy, or ACT, is a type of psychotherapy that facilitates you to radically accept the difficulties that come while living life in a valued direction. ACT is a form of mindfulness-based therapy, theorizing that greater well-being can be achieved by cognitively diffusing maladaptive thoughts and feelings. Essentially, ACT encourages the practice of here-and-now psychological flexibility, which helps reduce avoidant coping styles. ACT also tackles your commitment to making changes and allowing you to adhere to your goals and values.

To understand how these treatment approaches work, we must first dive deeply into the pool of anxiety disorders and how they can negatively impact your or a loved one's life. Towards the end of this chapter, we will transition how anxiety comes into play in a teenager's life.

According to Creswell et al. (2014), anxiety disorders are the most common psychiatric conditions in young people, with community studies that indicate a prevalence of 9% to 32% during childhood and adolescence. They have an explicit, adverse impact on educational achievement, family life, and leisure activities. These disorders may also be noticed with depression and behavioral disorders. There is a tangible probability that an anxious teenager will become an anxious adult and have impaired life outcomes. It is a cause for concern that, despite evidence-based interventions, most adolescents do not access treatment.

Therefore, it is important to recognize the early signs and symptoms of anxiety in a teenager and learn which type of anxiety they might have. Some of the most prevalent anxiety disorders in teens are classified as follows:

Specific Phobias

Fear about certain situations, activities, animals, or objects is relatively common. Fear is a rational response to problems that may threaten our safety.

However, certain people react to stimuli such as objects, activities, or situations irrationally exaggerating danger. Their feelings of panic, fear, or terror to these stimuli are entirely out of proportion to the actual threat. Sometimes, as little as a thought to the phobic stimulus may elicit a reaction. These excessive reactions are indicative of a specific phobia. Such people often know that their fear is irrational, but they consider it automatic or uncontrollable. Specific phobias occur in conjunction with panic attacks. Whereby a person might feel physical sensations like rapid heartbeat, choking, nausea, dizziness, chest pain, hot or cold flushes, and sweating. Psychological therapy and medications are the two treatment options available for such people.

Social Anxiety Disorder

Social Anxiety Disorder (SAD) is a recurrent, disproportionate fear of social situations where a person fears being criticized, judged, or even humiliated in front of others. It is not as simple as being shy or nervous in formal situations like public speaking, where someone might feel apprehensive. But it also happens in everyday cases, where eating in public, meeting people, or being watched while doing something becomes a horrific nuisance. A person may feel like they will embarrass themselves in such cases. This fear causes people to limit or avoid social situations, which strains their relationships, leading to loneliness, reduced academic capabilities or work accomplishments, depression, and substance abuse. Treatment includes psychological therapy to change your underlying thinking patterns and keep anxiety at bay. CBT and breathing exercises usually do the job, but sometimes antidepressants such as selective serotonin reuptake inhibitors (SSRIs) are needed.

Generalized Anxiety Disorder (GAD)

Generalized anxiety disorder is a type of anxiety disorder where people have persistent worry that interferes with their day-to-day life on an ongoing basis.

Such people have difficulty performing routine tasks. They have insomnia and constantly feel tense or restless. They have palpitations and dry mouths that cause them difficulty in speaking. They also have trouble concentrating and are often irritable. They have muscle tension, especially in their jaws or back. It is managed by psychological therapy or medicines.

Panic Disorder

This occurs when a person has frequent panic attacks, severely affecting their life. *A panic attack* is a response to a stressful situation where the sufferer feels like they are losing control. You might get a racing heartbeat, chest pain. You might also feel sweaty, shaky, dizzy, faint, and breathless. It is often mistaken for a heart attack because of the similar symptoms. *A panic disorder* is a compilation of frequent panic attacks where you constantly fear having one. You can undergo cognitive behavioral therapy, relaxation strategies, breathing exercises, mindfulness, meditation, and medication to manage a panic attack.

Agoraphobia

Agoraphobia is a kind of anxiety disorder where a person is terrified of having a panic attack in a public place such as a crowd or a queue where escaping from the situation is complicated. Such people avoid these situations and only agree to go to these places if someone accompanies them.

The triggers are usually stressful events, like losing a job or a relationship. The stressful event causes a person to be cut off from the outside world and gradually grow to include more places over time. This stressful event may also trigger a panic attack, so the sufferer will use any means necessary to avoid any situation that might trigger another attack.

It is treated by antidepressants, psychological therapy such as cognitive behavioral therapy (CBT), exposure therapy, education, counseling, and relaxation training.

Separation Anxiety

Separation anxiety is a specific phobia where separation from a parent or loved one generates overwhelming anxiety for the sufferer.

More than usual, separation anxiety is considered a disorder when it interferes with the person or their parent's life. It is regarded as a disorder if the person has more severe anxiety than their peers of the same age or if it prolongs consistently over at least four weeks. A panic attack may occur if the person is separated or even thinks about being separated from their loved one.

Treatment includes *exposure treatment* as a form of Cognitive Behavioral Therapy (CBT) that involves slowly increasing a person's ability to deal with their specific trigger.

Mood swings are inevitable among teens, and being a teenager is no easy job. Many teens struggle to find their identity and form relationships simultaneously, so they often face pressure at home and school. Add to that the added pressure that social media and the internet bring, and today's teens face the perfect storm of anxiety-inducing stimuli.

Adolescence can be stressful due to emotional demands and hormonal changes. Some teens express this turbulence with outbursts of anger, while others withdraw and refuse to tell their families what they're going through. Acting out or becoming isolated are considered behavioral problems when they are symptoms of heightened anxiety or even depression. Often, they go hand in hand. A little anxiety is normal, but it can become crippling—this is what we must watch out for in our young individuals.

It's normal to feel anxious when you're at risk. Fears during childhood and adolescence happen constantly: societal acceptance and rejection, overthinking, academic pressure, and countless factors could lead to heightened anxiety in our adolescents and teens.

This could range from anything between life-altering anxiety and a negligent drop-in functionality, dependent on the personality type of a child or a teenager.

There's a difference between normal anxiety and anxiety disorders because anxiety disorders cause persistent, disproportionate, or distorted responses that make it hard to function.

Adolescence is when the brain undergoes a massive and spectacular redesign to transition from dependent little people to independent, productive, happy adults.

The teen years can be fun and exciting, but many horrors exist. Adolescence can be filled with wonderful experiences, exciting discoveries, and gut-wrenching lows.

Walking the path to adulthood means that sometimes our kids feel like they're falling between the smaller, safer, more predictable world they've been used to and the more extensive, demanding, noisier world they're finding themselves in now.

As they get closer to adulthood - which will happen sometime in their early 20s - they might feel the ground beneath them is shaky.

There's often hard to separate regular emotional changes that come with puberty from anxiety that needs professional help.

Teenagers experience anxious feelings, affecting their ability to explore relationships, among other things, in ways that rob them of essential adolescent opportunities.

A young person's anxiety disorder can affect all aspects of their life, including their physical health, emotional well-being, and social skills. Because of the combined impact, they can feel socially isolated, stigmatized, and incapable of being active members of society.

A child's psychological well-being is directly related to their physical well-being. Both influence their thinking, feeling, and acting.

This book is for you if you want to lead a confident, independent, and happy life. If your anxiety is getting in the way of your hopes and dreams for the future, this book is your solution to combat all those problems!

Teen Anxiety: Drop the Rope is a survival guide demonstrating how CBT-based skills and mindfulness techniques can help you deal with your anxiety. It will give you the tools to change your thoughts, behaviors, and physical reactions toward anxiety through simple and practical exercises.

CHAPTER 2:

ANXIETY AND TEENS

We all remember what it feels like to be a teenager.

A rush of hormones.

A surge of emotions.

The familiar feeling of being misunderstood by everyone.

It's like juggling too many things at once and often dropping them.

Buried under a constant burden to perform well at schoolwork, managing a social media identity, fretting about career plans, bullying, sexism, racism, physical appearance, love life, peer pressure, meeting parents' expectations, and competing with siblings for attention. And in most cases, this is not even the tip of the iceberg.

And you know what's the worst part?

An average teenager cannot escape their problems at all. There is always a constant reminder lurking in the background, telling them they aren't good enough or aren't doing enough. The hyper connections of social media chase the teenager of today until they fall into the sinkhole.

As discussed in the previous chapter, anxiety is the most common mental health disorder in the United States, affecting nearly one-third of both adolescents, according to the National Institute of Mental Health. Unlike depression, with which it routinely occurs, in light of consensus, anxiety often takes a backseat as a less severe mental health problem.

"Anxiety is easy to dismiss or overlook, partially because everyone has it to some degree," explained Philip Kendall, director of the Child and Adolescent Anxiety Disorders Clinic at Temple University in Philadelphia. "It has an evolutionary purpose; it helps us detect and avoid potentially dangerous situations. Highly anxious people, though, have an overactive fightorflight response that perceives threats where there often are none".

We must remember that at this delicate stage of life, along with social, physical, and emotional changes, teenagers are subjected to rapidly changing brains.

This brain remodeling happens intensively during adolescence, continuing until the child is in their mid-20s. Brain changes depend heavily on age, experience, and hormonal changes in puberty.

The unused connections in the *thinking* and *processing* part of your child's brain (the grey matter) are pruned away. Simultaneously, other relationships are strengthened. This is called the *"use it or lose it"* principle and is the brain's way of becoming efficient.

This pruning process begins in the back of the brain. The front part of the brain, the prefrontal cortex, is remodeled last. The prefrontal cortex is the decision-making part of the brain, responsible for a child's ability to plan and think about the consequences of actions, solve problems, and control impulses. Changes in this part of the brain continue into early adulthood.

Because the prefrontal cortex is still developing, teenagers might rely on the part of the brain called the amygdala to make decisions and solve problems more than adults do. The amygdala is associated with emotions, impulses, aggression, and instinctive behavior.

This is why sometimes a child's thinking and behavior seem relatively mature, whereas other times, the child might seem to behave illogically or impulsively and have emotional outbursts. The back-to-front development of the brain is responsible for this, so you might say that teenagers are working with brains still under construction.

The amalgamation of each child's unique brain development and environment makes up for how they feel, act, and think. Teenage is the crucial time when certain behaviors and skills might become *hardwired* in the brain.

While the brain is still developing, teens might demonstrate risky behavior, express strong emotions, and become prone to impulsive decision-making.

As a parent or caregiver, you can curtail this by encouraging positive behavior patterns, promoting good thinking skills, and helping them get plenty of sleep and leisure time.

Cognitive behavioral therapy (CBT) is one of the most influential and widely used psychosocial treatments for teen-related anxiety. In CBT, therapists help individuals with anxiety to gradually and repeatedly expose themselves to the situations they fear.

Practicing something that causes fear or anxiety can lessen its power in real-life situations.

A socially anxious teen might start by imagining sending a classmate a text asking to hang out, gradually move on to sending that text, or even calling a classmate on the phone, and eventually initiating a conversation with an unfamiliar peer at a party. The goal is to practice these anxiety-provoking actions and associate them with a new state of safety.

Decades of studies in animals and humans have helped psychology researchers understand more about how the brain regulates fear.

Building on this work, emerging neuroscience evidence suggests that current treatments for anxiety directly modify the same amygdala-prefrontal connections that are in flux during adolescence and implicated in anxiety.

Anxiety is a rational reaction to unstable, dangerous circumstances for many young people, particularly those raised in abusive families or who live in neighborhoods besieged by poverty or violence.

Their families are not safe, and neither are their neighborhoods or streets. They often come from backgrounds with a history of trauma or abuse.

In these economically disadvantaged communities, teens who *act out* are frequently labeled defiant and aggressive, and teens who *keep to themselves* are called silent sufferers or mistaken for being shy and often overlooked.

In contrast, teenagers who are raised in more affluent communities might seemingly have less to feel anxious about. But Suniya Luthar, a professor of psychology at Arizona State University who has studied resilience and distress in both prosperous and disadvantaged teenagers, has identified that privileged youths are among the most emotionally distressed people in America.

These teens are incredibly anxious and perfectionistic, but they are often dealt with scorn and contempt because of their economic condition.

For several teens, the pressure is relentless and worsens over time. Their most significant stressor is that they never get to a point where they can say I've done enough or performed enough; they always keep going.

Anxious teens certainly existed before social media. But the digital habits of today's teens, round-the-clock responding to texts, posting to social media, and obsessively following the filtered exploits of peers, are to blame for their anxiety. It drastically affects their moods and personalities and is a tool they can't survive without, silently obliterating their mental health. Their tortured relationship with social media is tied to their self-worth.

Smartphones not only provoke anxiety but serve as an avoidance strategy for teens. These help them create an "illusion of control and certainty, "which is how they desperately try to manage their environments.

In real-world situations, this predictability is useless because they must interact in socially awkward situations and learn by trial and error how to survive them.

Adolescents with anxiety are hypervigilant. They are typically tense and on guard. They scan their environments for signs of perceived danger and are reactive to slight environmental changes because of heightened sensitivity to threats. Compared with nonanxious adolescents, they are more likely to selectively attend to threatening information and interpret more information in a situation as threatening.

Scientifically put, American Psychiatric Association, 2000, says that *avoidance* is a hallmark of all anxiety disorders, especially social anxiety disorder. Avoidance is not just a behavioral act but has undertones of cognitive recognition of a situation as threatening or dangerous. Avoidance is also a trait that is not only exclusive to anxiety but may overlap with a mood disorder like depression.

Rumination, or the focus and rethinking of thoughts about a negative situation, is most often associated with depressive symptoms. Garnefski and Kraaij (2006) found that rumination was one of the components of emotional regulation strongly related to depressive symptoms.

Understanding these two concepts is integral when discussing teen anxiety because anxious behaviors if left unregulated, can become more sinister.

If left untreated, anxiety disorders can lead to episodes of clinical depression and hinder their academic performance. They can also increase teenagers' chances of resorting to drugs and alcohol to alleviate anxiety symptoms.

When someone with anxiety has a panic attack or experiences symptoms like anger, irritability, or fear, it triggers an internal chemical cascade similar to the *flight or fight response*. Once this reflex kicks in, the brain signals the endocrine system to release the cortisol stress hormone.

This thunderstorm of cortisol in the blood in an acute or short-term scenario is necessary for our feedback mechanism. But in the case of chronic stress or an anxiety disorder, our bodies are not programmed to deal with this cortisol flood.

Chronic exposure to cortisol can directly cause or exacerbate high blood pressure, decrease immune responses, and lead to heart disease, obesity, and chronic fatigue.

To summarize, hypervigilance, reactivity to new or changes in stimuli, hypersensitivity to threats, avoidant coping, somatic complaints, catastrophic reactions, and excessive parent accommodation can collectively be helpful indicators that anxiety may be present among teenagers.

Anxiety is treatable, and there is hope.

According to the latest research, the integrated treatment model is the best treatment for teen anxiety. The integrated model for teen anxiety typically means a mix of psychotherapy and, in some cases, medication.

During treatment, a teen with anxiety can learn practical tools to manage their symptoms. When they learn to manage their symptoms, they can reduce or eliminate the consequences of untreated anxiety. First, they're getting treatment, and second, because you, as the parent or caregiver, validate their real mental health disorder experience.

You can support creating a healthy foundation by providing your teen with healthy meals with whole grains, fresh fruits, and vegetables and helping them develop an exercise routine to get their body moving and blood flowing. Encouraging them to spend time outdoors, at least an hour to spend in nature. Monitor their sleeping schedule and make sure they get at least 8-10 hours of uninterrupted sleep each night. Limit their sugar and caffeine intake since these can act as triggers.

In the next chapter, you will learn how to identify the signs and symptoms of anxiety. But once you create the foundation for positive mental health by making sure you contribute to healthy behaviors, rest assured, your teen will have an affinity with their mental health professional and work synergistically to guarantee positive treatment outcomes and overall well-being.

CHAPTER 3:

SPOTTING THE SIGNS

Picture this:

Alex is an average 14-year-old from a humble household. He goes to public school and performs well academically. Suddenly, his mother gets diagnosed with terminal cancer. At first, his parents try to hide the news from him, thinking it is in his best interest. But he overhears them making appointments with specialists and often catches his mother crying while doing routine tasks. He notices her deteriorating health and finds himself powerless to help her. It triggers feelings of rage and hopelessness in him.

He tries to confront his parents about this tragic news but doesn't know how. Instead, he withdraws from them. He starts to show little or no interest in attending school. His grades start to suffer, and he finds any excuse to escape social interactions. He stays in bed longer than usual and begins to ignore his personal hygiene. He plays with the food on his plate at mealtimes and justifies it to his parents by saying he had snacked at school earlier. This causes him to lose weight and become lethargic. He keeps to his room, playing video games in isolation and conversing with his family. He also loses his temper and aggressively breaks things around the house.

Concerned about this drastic onset of behavioral change, his parents sit him down and break the news to him. He tells them he is already aware of his mother's disease and feels betrayed that they would not trust him enough to say to him. He finally lets his guard down and is reduced to tears, unable to hide his emotions for a change. His parents console him and decide to consult a psychologist to deal with his suffering.

The scenario above explains an adolescent who cannot process his feelings about facing the illness and the possibility of losing a parent. He cannot navigate his emotional turmoil and exhibits erratic behavior as a response to the trigger.

As a parent or caregiver, you must be vigilant to such signs of *acting out* and know when it is time for professional intervention.

If you have made the simple effort of *spotting the signs*, then well done! Pat yourself on the back because that is the first step on the way to the recovery of your child.

The emotional outbursts on the part of your teenager are a cry for help. They are not to be overlooked. If left undiagnosed, they could become a plethora of mental illnesses ranging from harmless misconduct to more sinister problems like depression.

What started as social withdrawals could morph into behaviors that negatively affect a teenager's education and severely stunt the development of critical social relationships. This will consequentially take a disastrous toll on their lifestyle and, more importantly, their mental and physical health.

Finding out your teen is dealing with anxiety can be a frightening experience. Your mind starts to race with self-criticism, often unwarranted and harsh.

Where did I go wrong? Will this go away by itself? Is this going to affect my teen long-term?

At this moment, you must ensure you do not lose sight of what is essential.

Treatments are available, and recovery is possible!

This book will guide you to decide against seeking professional help because you must remember that a timely diagnosis promises successful treatment outcomes.

When it comes to anxiety, anxious teens are different from anxious children. Younger children often worry about things like the dark, monsters, or something terrible happening to their parents. But teenagers are more likely to be concerned about themselves.

This behavior is habitually hidden under the guise of perfectionism. Teens fear not performing well in school or sports. They can also be worried about their appearance or how people perceive them. Going through the sensitive puberty stage triggers worries about their bodies, and a comparison to their peers is not uncommon.

Noticing changes in children and teens is crucial, as symptoms of most mental health challenges start before age 25. Addressing these concerns as soon as possible is critical: The quicker we address the problem, the better chance a young person can return to everyday activities.

Anxiety disorders can affect every part of a young person's life, including physical health, emotional well-being, and social skill development. The combined impact can make teens feel socially isolated, stigmatized, and incapable of being active community members.

Mental health has a direct relationship with a child's physical health. Both physical and psychological health influence how teens think, feel, and act on both the inside and out.

Sometimes, as a parent or caregiver, it might be challenging to notice anxiety or spot variations in behavior because teens hide their feelings exceptionally well. Instead of accepting their emotions, they often lash out at the people around them. They could also start to complain about experiencing physical symptoms like stomach aches or headaches. They may even resort to drugs to drown out their feelings. This is their catharsis of sorts.

There is substantial evidence that the pandemic has increased the number of adolescents that suffer from anxiety. With frequent lockdowns, social distancing, isolation from friends, and fluctuating educational schedules, covid has shaken teenage mental health to its core.

Teenagers are not impervious to environmental variations, and instability only exacerbates anxious behavior.

Students with anxiety disorders are easily frustrated; they may have difficulty completing their work. They may worry so much about getting everything right that they take much longer to finish than other students. Or they may refuse to begin out of fear that they won't be able to do anything properly.

Their fear of embarrassment, humiliation, or failure may result in school avoidance. Getting behind in their work due to numerous absences often creates a vicious cycle of fear of failure, increased anxiety, and avoidance, which leads to more absences. Teens who have undergone trauma may have difficulty concentrating on work, as they are focused on the traumatic event and ensuring they can avoid it.

They may also be distracted frequently by reminders of the trauma triggering 'flashbacks,' leading to an inability to complete work. Their reactions may be out of context given the current situation as they react to their perception of events or reminders of past events.

Reminders may come from any of the senses and may seem innocuous to others (e.g., the smell of a person, the rustle of leaves, the touch of a friend, or the use of a particular word). Without an obvious trigger, emotional reactions may be fear, horror, anger, or hopelessness. Younger teens are not likely to identify anxious feelings, which may make it difficult for parents to understand the reason behind poor school performance fully.

Your child may be shy. The two differ while shy teens may be more likely to feel socially anxious. Being introverted does not cause extreme anxiety or panic in a social environment. Shyness, in addition, is a part of a child's personality. Social anxiety is a fear of embarrassment in a social situation that causes avoidance. You must not confuse the two.

Remember!

People can't just snap out of being anxious. Anxiety is not a light switch that can be flipped on and off. While the behavior of a nervous teen may seem trivial to you-trust me when I say this- it is not insignificant to them!

Since the cycle of anxiety and avoidance feeds off itself, you must never discredit your teen's feelings or changes in behavior because, more often than not, an anxiety-ridden teen needs help from a parent and a professional to break this cycle.

Teens struggling with anxiety, particularly social anxiety disorder, often choose to isolate themselves. They do so to avoid the stress of interacting with others.

Social withdrawal often ends up feeding anxiety even more. An isolated person becomes more internalized. This causes them to focus on negative thoughts.

Anxiety can interfere with a person's ability to see the world from someone else's perspective. As a result, anxiety sufferers may also experience difficulty creating new empathetic bonds.

See if you notice any significant shifts in your child's social habits. Some indicative behavior is:

Fewer interactions with friends

Skipping extracurricular activities

Spending more time alone than usual

Realize this, sufferers of anxiety need distractions. It's complicated for someone to overcome fear on their own.

According to John Piacentini, Ph.D. and Lindsey Bergman, Ph.D., from the UCLA Child Anxiety Resilience Education and Support Centre, you should be wary of the following signs in your teenager,

Physical signs of anxiety

Often complains of headaches or stomachaches, with no medical reason

Refuses to eat in the school cafeteria or other public places

Changes in eating habits suddenly

Won't use restrooms away from home

Gets restless, fidgety, hyperactive, or distracted (but doesn't necessarily have ADHD)

Starts to shake or sweat in intimidating situations

Constantly tenses muscles

Has developed coping mechanisms like fidgeting, nail-biting, messing with their hair, tapping hands or feet, head nodding, frustrated or hesitated breathing. Lip biting, sweaty palms, racing heartbeat, and trembling hands

Has trouble falling asleep or staying asleep

Emotional signs of anxiety

Frequent crying episodes

Becomes cranky or angry for no clear reason

Is afraid of making even minor mistakes

Has extreme test anxiety

Doubts their skills and abilities, even when there's no reason to

Can't handle any criticism, no matter how constructive

Has panic attacks (or is afraid of having panic attacks)

Has pressing fears or phobias

Worries about things way off in the future

Often has nightmares about losing a parent or loved one

Has obsessive thoughts or concerns about bad things happening or upsetting topics

Behavioral signs of anxiety

Avoids participating in class activities

Stays silent or preoccupied when expected to work with others

Refuses to go to school or do schoolwork

Avoids social situations with peers

Refuses to speak to peers or strangers in stores, restaurants, etc.

Becomes emotional or angry when separating from family or loved ones

Begins to have explosive outbursts

Starts withdrawing from activities

Constantly seeks approval from parents, teachers, and friends

Has compulsive behaviors, like frequent

handwashing or arranging things

To recap, the onset of anxiety may be fulminant, but you should be on the lookout for some characteristic symptoms of anxiety. They are recurring fear and worry, trouble concentrating, self-consciousness or sensitivity to criticism, social withdrawal, and avoidance.

Once you develop the necessary observational skills for the fluctuations in your teen's behavior, they will be conducive to identifying patterns and conducting regular mental health checks with a professional for a prompt diagnosis and fruitful treatment.

CHAPTER 4:

WHY DOES IT HAPPEN?

"I believe that everything happens for a reason. People change so that you can learn to let go, things go wrong so that you appreciate them when they're right, you believe lies so you eventually learn to trust no one but yourself, and sometimes good things fall apart so better things can fall together."

-Marilyn Monroe

You must have heard the axiom "everything happens for a reason" multiple times. So, how does it apply to the human condition?

Well, in the words of Aristotle, the universe is in a state of constant motion—constantly changing and always evolving. However, what remains, remains constant is what Aristotle termed *Entelechy*.

Entelechy is your "unique to you" highest potential. He said that everything and everyone on this planet possessed this unique potential. And not only does each being have this potential, but they also can grow into this potential and harness it to their benefit.

Even a mighty tree starts as a seedling. It weathers every rain and storm that it encounters to become what it is destined to be.

Similarly, you can tap into your adversities to grow into your highest and mightiest self. You can mobilize your innate abilities or, as put by Aristotle, your *conscious insight* to reach that final form.

There is always a purpose, meaning, and growth waiting to be gained from whatever affliction you face. You are one step closer to a happier life if you consistently tap into your entelechy or your conscious insight and never lose sight of your life's purpose on this asteroid we call Earth.

Whatever storms might come your way, you should never preoccupy yourself with the why but rather ponder where the events take you. And know in your heart that this place, where you are supposed to be, is somewhere better and more beautiful from where you started. And once you get to that place, you will understand why you had to go through all those difficult times, and the transformation you will inculcate in yourself will be worth all the wait!

If this still reads as convoluted to you, then don't worry. Let me explain *why (reasons for your/your teen's anxiety)* so you might appreciate the *when (your recovery)*.

Etiology of Anxiety

Adolescence is a sensitive time to navigate self-identity and pressure from every angle, but have you wondered why some teens find it difficult to thrive and suffer from anxiety and depression while others don't?

Cabral and Patel (2020) note that adolescents with maladaptive responses to everyday situations and stressors are at risk of having anxiety disorders. Persistent anxiety symptoms and disorders can be debilitating, with long-term adverse outcomes in adulthood. We must first understand the etiology to decrease the burden of anxiety disorders.

The development of anxiety disorders has a multifactorial etiology. There is a considerable complex interaction of genetics, temperament, parenting behavior, environmental triggers, and physiologic factors. Identifying these risk factors is vital to early detection, prevention, and development of applicable management approaches.

Genetics

Studies by Lazary et al. (2019) show that adults with version FAAH C385A of the FAAH gene reportedly have less anxiety and exhibit an aberration in brain connections than those with anxiety. This marked difference is in their prefrontal cortex, which is more tightly wired to the deeper parts of the brain where emotional memories are stored.

They examined data from 1,050 healthy participants, ages 3-21, including their genotype, psychological assessments, and brain scans. They found that those with the protective C385A allele showed higher frontal limbic connectivity and lower self-reported anxiety, but only after 12 years.

In children younger than 12, the gene didn't have noticeable anxiety effects. That indicates that the changes in gene activity over time may lead to the development of anxiety disorders.

Understanding the variety of genes that influence brain wiring and function is a promising feat for developing tailored treatments for anxiety sufferers in the future.

UNC Health psychiatric epidemiologist Dr. Anna Bauer, Ph.D., MPH, suggests that children of parents diagnosed with anxiety disorder are seven times more likely to develop an anxiety disorder.

Genetics combined with environmental factors such as a parent's behavior or traumatic events can create the conditions for anxiety to manifest.

So, what exactly runs in the family is the risk of developing these disorders combined with an inviting environment.

We are born with our genetic code, but our environment influences the expression of anxiety genes. Dr. Bauer explains that anxiety is thought to be about 30% inherited but is exacerbated by environmental factors such as learned behaviors or stressful situations.

Environment

Teenagers' social, school, and home environments can impact their mental health.

Difficulties such as abuse, neglect, family divorce, bullying, poverty, learning disabilities, and struggling to fit in contribute to anxiety.

From getting good grades, choosing the right career path, and having an impressive application form good enough to get into the college of their choice, academic pressure and school-related stress are severe contributors to many students' anxiety. So many teenagers nowadays have to juggle school with part-time jobs and extracurricular activities (such as student governments, after-school sports, and volunteer work).

On top of that, they are also expected to maintain active social lives *and* good grades by studying, doing homework, and turning in many projects. Such a hectic schedule leaves little time for relaxation.

Consequently, most teenagers don't get the proper amount of sleep, neglect their self-care, and deal with high levels of chronic stress on a day-to-day basis – all of which exacerbate feelings of anxiety (Putwain, 2007).

In his research, Twenge (2019) notes that Between 2011 and 2018, rates of depression, self-harm, and suicide attempts increased substantially among U.S. adolescents who used technology.

The most probable causes of these trends likely 1) began or accelerated during these years, 2) affected many people, 3) impacted everyday life, and 4) were associated with depression.

In several extensive studies, heavy technology users are twice as likely as light users to be depressed or have low well-being. They are associated with declines in happiness and life satisfaction and increases in depression and suicide attempts.

Social media also creates a culture of constant distraction that teenagers escape to when they feel bored, lonely, or upset, which stunts their emotional growth and keeps them from developing healthy coping mechanisms and mental resilience (White, 2013).

Tianchu Han, in 2021, cited that with the containment of the COVID-19 pandemic becoming normality, adolescent anxiety and mental illnesses increasingly emerge on a global scale.

He explains that even teenagers raised in a reasonably favorable background suffer from mental issues relating to environmental changes due to the pandemic.

He attributes these changes to family conflicts, online studying, and lack of social contact overall.

Parents concerned about passing on anxiety can't change their children's genes, but they can work to create a less anxious environment.

Anxious families tend to overestimate negative information, so if a worried parent responds to tragic news on social media, they are less likely to let their children go out in the world where they might be exposed to harm.

As parents, you must realize that you might be modeling anxious beliefs and behaviors for your children. They mimic and do what they have inherited and absorbed from you.

If you are a parent struggling with anxiety, getting yourself into therapy will immensely benefit your children.

In their study, Ebbert et al., 2019, state that as children move through adolescence, their attachment to their parents changes significantly, with the most significant drop occurring in middle school. Attachment levels stabilized by the end of high school, but the more a teen felt alienated during adolescence, the less likely they were to trust and communicate with their parents.

It would be helpful if, during this time of adolescence, parents would look past all the moodiness, distance, and irritability and express feelings of love and affirmation.

The study involved 335 children in 6th grade in 1998 who lived in an affluent white-collar community. Each of the children was given an annual assessment until they were 18 years old, which asked them to rate their attachment to their mothers and fathers and their levels of anxiety and depression.

They found that higher rates of emotional alienation from parents were linked to more emotional problems. Preteens, specifically, felt over one-and-a-half times as alienated in middle school as they did at an earlier age, and they reported a threefold decrease in trust. As a result, communication dropped about four times as much.

Teens who felt more alienated and lost trust in their mothers (more so than fathers) were more likely to have high anxiety levels by 12th grade. This held true for depression as well.

The more communication increased by the end of high school, the more likely the teen was to experience symptoms of depression.

Parents can protect their teens' mental health if at least one of them has a strong, supportive relationship with the teen.

For parents to be there for their children, they must look after themselves first.

Remember, you can't pour from an empty cup!

Trauma

A traumatic experience is any event in life that causes a threat to our safety and potentially places our own life or the lives of others at risk. As a result, a person experiences high levels of emotional, psychological, and physical distress that temporarily disrupts their ability to function normally in day-to-day life.

These strong emotions often concern teenagers who experience a distressing or frightening event. Even though these reactions usually subside as a part of the body's natural healing and recovery process, parents or caregivers must understand how a teenager manages distress and trauma to support and help the young person.

Teenagers can also be distraught by local, national, or international tragedies or trauma that affects their friends. Your teenager will handle trauma differently than younger children or adults. Younger child depends directly on their family, whereas many teenagers look to their peer group for support. To help them, parents need to understand how teenagers manage distress.

Teenagers with a history of trauma, such as sexual abuse, violence, or involvement in an accident, may be more likely to experience anxiety and depression.

School shootings, sexual assault, kidnappings, hazing, and other violent, heinous crimes make the world seem like a terrifying place to live in, especially for teenagers.

Exposure to such violence can make young people anxious about being alone in public places, going out, and walking home late at night. Many don't even feel safe in their cities or neighborhoods because of how rampant crime is nowadays. And these feelings of helplessness and dread can leave teens overwhelmed with anxiety and fear for their own safety.

Martin et al. (2014) postulate that stressful life events in adolescents have been found to be directly proportional to higher anxiety sensitivity.

When a child or an adult is threatened, the person's stress response system will be activated, triggering the sympathetic nervous system's fight or flight response. The impact of early and/or chronic trauma can be far-reaching and sometimes span a lifetime.

Researchers believe that there are sensitive periods for the development of specific capabilities. These developmental windows of opportunity allow certain brain parts to be available for particular types of growth.

According to Perry (2009), brain development in infancy and early childhood lays the foundation for all future development. Neural pathways form at great speed and depend on the repetition of experiences.

Experiences teach the brain what to expect and how to respond. When experiences are traumatic, the pathways getting the most use are those in response to the trauma; this reduces the formation of other pathways needed for adaptive behavior.

Three areas of the brain whose function may be altered in response to chronic and extraordinary trauma have been identified: the prefrontal cortex, amygdala, and hippocampus. In human studies, the amygdala is intensely involved in the formation of emotional memories, especially fear-related memories (Applegate and Shapiro, 2005)

There appears to be a neurophysiologic dysfunction in the emotion regulation in amygdala-prefrontal circuitry in individuals who were emotionally abused as children. These disorders are associated with dysfunction within myriad amygdala-based networks throughout the prefrontal cortex. Without treatment, repeated childhood exposure to traumatic events can affect the brain and nervous system and increase health-risk behaviors (e.g., smoking, eating disorders, substance use, and other high-risk activities).

When teens experience trauma, they can begin to feel helpless because the trauma can invade and affect any aspect of a teen's life. Trauma in teens is associated with higher rates of depression and anxiety and lower academic achievement.

Teens are also more likely than other age groups to engage in risky behaviors after traumatic experiences. They don't always know that they can turn to adults for help, continuing to struggle alone and even lashing out when parents and other adults reach out.

A teenager may have breakdowns in communication because of being deeply upset by a traumatic event. They often may not want to share their feelings with their parents. They become aloof and appear strong in front of their family members. In most cases, they prefer to discuss it with their peers.

Problems may worsen if

The family doesn't talk about the event.

The family misunderstands the teenager's behavior and assumes the teenager is just being difficult or taking advantage of the situation.

Parents try to keep the teenager from their peer group or criticize their choice of friends.

Parents feel hurt or angry because the teenager prefers to talk to friends about the event rather than the family.

The family argues over different points of view

Parents try to get emotional support from the teenager.

Substance Abuse

Teen anxiety and substance abuse issues are firmly connected, as drugs and alcohol are commonly used to self-medicate symptoms like anxiety.

Teenagers are already prone to impulsive, risky, and dangerous behaviors. Abusing substances makes these potentially hazardous behaviors more likely. Since a teen's brain is still developing and growing, the brain is receiving and retaining information as the teen grows. This means the brain will learn from drugs and alcohol, affecting the brain's processes. As a result, the teen will miss many opportunities to learn new skills. Many teens experience a significant deficit in their cognitive functions, impairing their ability to learn and perform well in school. Substance abuse will interfere with a teen's logical thinking, rationality, and ability to weigh negative consequences. Some of the other effects of teen substance abuse can include:

Car accidents	Assaults
Unplanned pregnancies	Damaged relationships

Delayed or missed educational opportunities

Violent behavior

Sexually transmitted diseases

Poor hygiene

Depression

Loss of interest

Emotional problems

Delinquent behavior

Teen anxiety and substance abuse disorders are interlinked because struggling with a mental health condition increases the risk of developing psychological or physical dependency. While drugs and alcohol may momentarily alleviate anxiety, substances ultimately aggravate mental health disorders. Addiction causes significant neurotransmitter imbalances. Often, mental health conditions link to neurotransmitter abnormalities. Thus, addiction can worsen mental health symptoms.

Teen anxiety and substance abuse problems can aggravate symptoms, and worsened anxiety symptoms can lead sufferers to use more substances to self-medicate.

Another complication of teen anxiety and substance abuse disorders is that having a co-occurring condition makes recovery more difficult. The complex relationship between mental health and addiction means that dual diagnosis programs are necessary because recovery requires treating symptoms of both disorders to recover fully.

Even if your teen receives treatment for an anxiety disorder while suffering from an addiction, substance abuse makes mental health medications ineffective. Taking medicines for an anxiety disorder while abusing drugs can also increase their risk of experiencing an overdose.

Stresses of puberty

Teenagers going through puberty are exposed to hormonal changes that affect their mood. They also undergo body changes, making them feel insecure or different from their peers.

Your teen's hormone production ebbs and flows during adolescence. Sometimes your teen might feel anxious, upset, depressed, and angry for no reason. Hormonal fluctuations likely cause some of this. Teenage boys are dealing with testosterone surges, and adolescent girls are dealing with hormonal shifts due to menstruation; combined with a lack of experience in dealing with these feelings and general immaturity, hormones are a recipe for stress and teenage anxiety.

Kids today are under much pressure from their peers. Peer pressure can be positive or negative, but both types raise stress levels. For example, being pressured to shoplift or commit some other crime is stressful and an example of negative peer pressure.

If your teen's peers are all getting excellent grades, applying to good universities, and dating the football or cheerleading team captain, this puts much pressure on your teen to conform and keep up.

Another type of anxiety that peers exacerbate is social anxiety. Your teen might dread going to school and talking to people. This condition can be caused by bullying, or it can just appear seemingly out of nowhere.

Negative thought patterns

Depression and anxiety in teenagers may be linked to negative thought patterns. If teenagers have regular exposure to negative thinking, often from their parents, they may develop a pessimistic worldview.

Teens with mental health disorders are especially critical of themselves. They can get stuck in negative thinking patterns that contribute to depression, amp up their anxiety, or make painful emotions feel overwhelming.

If your studious teen cannot perform in a specific exam, they may think they are not good enough and will do even worse in the next exam. If your teen forgets a line in a school play, they may think they ruined the performance.

These negative thinking patterns are often unrealistic but can significantly impact our emotions, behaviors, and worldviews. Mental health experts call them cognitive distortions, sometimes called cognitive errors, thinking mistakes, or thinking errors.

Now, it is normal for a human to make mistakes. When that kind of thinking is chronic and entrenched, the thoughts likely affect a child's emotional life.

Negative thinking patterns are often a sign of rumination (overthinking). Rumination changes the brain's hardwiring: we all have negative thoughts, but not all fall into negative thinking patterns.

Let us discuss the types of negative thinking patterns:

All or Nothing

The All or Nothing thought pattern doesn't operate on a spectrum. In fact, like with most negative thought patterns, things are very black and white. For teens struggling with this thought pattern, either everything is going very well, or it's all going south. A teen struggling with this thought pattern might use absolute terms like *never* or *always*.

An example of this thought pattern might be that your teen doesn't get into the soccer team they wanted to be a part of, so your teen tells you, "I'll never try out for this soccer again. It's over."

Fortune Telling

With this thought pattern, your teen predicts things that can happen, and these predictions are most often negative.

For example, "I don't want to go to college because I'll fail anyway." Another example would be, "I don't want to go to the party because I'm going to do something embarrassing, and people will laugh at me."

Negative Self-Label & Personalization

As the term implies, with negative self-labels, your teen cannot differentiate negative occurrences from themselves.

For example, if your teen doesn't get the text from a friend they've been waiting for, they might think things like, "He didn't text me because he doesn't like me," or "They didn't talk to me because I'm weird."

Minimizing

With minimizing, your teen might not see all the good things happening around them, or they might not truly appreciate the good and healthy things in their lives. Your teen cannot celebrate their accomplishments or the good things around them.

For example, after getting a good grade on a test, your teen might tell you something like, "Well, I didn't study for it. I'm just lucky."

Mind Reading

This is when your teen assumes that they know and understand what another person is thinking, typically being sure it reflects poorly on them.

For example, I'm talking, and the person I'm talking to doesn't seem to be paying attention. I'm sure they don't like me. (In fact, it might be that they're just distracted or stressed about something unrelated to you and are having difficulty focusing.)

Catastrophizing

(also called Magnification)

This is when a teen takes a problem or something negative and blows it up out of proportion.

For example, This party is going to be the worst experience ever! Or: If I don't get a high SAT score, I'll die of embarrassment.

Mental Filter(also called Selective Abstraction)

This is essentially seeing only the negative instead of looking at all the positive or neutral aspects of an experience.

For example, your teen writes a paper for a teacher, giving them plenty of positive feedback on it, but they spelled someone's name wrong. They can only think about the misspelling for the rest of the day.

Personalization

Making things about them when they are not. This includes blaming themselves for what is beyond their control and taking things personally when they are not intended to harm them.

For example: If I hadn't demanded so much of my parents, maybe they wouldn't get divorced. Or: How dare that person walk before me — that was so disrespectful!

Imperatives

Thinking in "shoulds" and "musts" (and the inverse, "should nots" and must not").

For example, I should be able to give presentations in class without feeling any anxiety. What's wrong with me?

These negative thought patterns are diverse and have different roots and ways of presenting themselves. In the upcoming chapters, I will help you understand the use of strategies like Cognitive Behavioral Therapy or CBT to manage and eradicate them.

To sum it up, in this chapter, you learned about the multifactorial expression of anxiety in teens and the role of these causes in the behavioral psychology of your teen.

In the following chapters, you will learn how to identify and manage these causes and practice techniques to alleviate them entirely. You will also know when to seek professional help. You will learn about the treatment modalities available, their pros and cons, and which one fits you best.

Remember, do not discontinue the search prematurely or get discouraged when approaching a therapist who is not a good fit. You will find help that caters to you, I promise.

So, keep on reading!

CHAPTER 5:

PERSON-CENTERED APPROACH

'When the other person is hurting, confused, troubled, anxious, alienated, terrified; or when he or she is doubtful of self-worth, uncertain as to identity, then understanding is called for. The gentle and sensitive companionship of an empathic stance… provides illumination and healing. In such situations, deep understanding is, I believe, the most precious gift one can give to another." —Carl R. Rogers

This quote perfectly captures the essence of the Person-Centered Approach. In this chapter, we'll explore the fundamental principles of this approach and discuss its potential benefits for young people struggling with anxious thoughts and feelings.

We'll also share some real-life stories and examples to help illustrate how the Person-Centered Approach works in practice.

The Person-Centered Approach is also known as Client-Centered Therapy. This approach was developed by Carl Rogers, one of the most influential psychologists of the 20th century, and it has been used successfully to treat a wide range of mental health conditions, including anxiety.

Rogers believed that when people struggle with emotional distress, such as anxiety, they need empathic understanding and compassionate support.

In treating teenage anxiety, this means that when a teenager feels overwhelmed by anxious thoughts and emotions, they need someone to listen to them with kindness and empathy, without judgment or criticism.

This is exactly what a Person-Centered therapist aims to provide—a safe and non-judgmental space where teenagers can explore their feelings and thoughts.

The therapist can help the teenager feel heard and understood by offering empathic companionship, creating a sense of validation and acceptance.

This can be a decisive first step towards healing and growth as the teenager begins to feel more comfortable exploring their inner experiences and build greater self-awareness and self-compassion.

As Rogers noted, "In such situations, deep understanding is, I believe, the most precious gift one can give to another." By offering this gift of understanding and empathy, a Person-Centered therapist can help a teenager to build greater resilience and coping skills, which can ultimately help them to manage their anxiety more effectively.

Believing strongly that theory should come out of practice rather than the other way round, Rogers developed his theory based on his work with emotionally troubled people and claimed that we have a remarkable capacity for self-healing and personal growth leading towards self-actualization. He emphasized the person's current perception and how we live here and now.

Rogers noticed that people describe their current experiences by referring to themselves in some way, for example, "I don't understand what's happening" or "I feel different to how I used to feel."

Central to Rogers' (1959) theory is the notion of self or self-concept. This is *"the organized, consistent set of perceptions and beliefs about oneself."*

It comprises all the ideas and values that characterize 'I' and 'me,' including perception and valuing of *'what I am'* and *'what I can do.'*

Let's ponder over the philosophy of what Rogers once said,

"The curious paradox is that when I accept myself just as I am, I can change."

This is the crux of our discussion on this revolutionary approach that embodies the benefits of self-acceptance in its visceral form.

Before the advent of humanistic therapies in the 1950s, the predominant therapeutic approaches were behavioral and psychodynamic, which emphasized clients' unconscious or subconscious experience rather than their conscious experiences and behaviors (McLeod, 2015).

While many of today's popular forms of therapy have shifted towards a more client-centered approach, a particular form of therapy stands out due to its strong emphasis on the client and its avoidance of providing any direct guidance or advice.

The Person-Centered Approach is characterized by its focus on providing a non-judgmental and empathic environment that empowers clients to explore their own experiences and find their solutions.

Before we dive into the mechanics of this specific form of therapy, let me expound upon the concept again with an anecdote for your better understanding.

Sophie was a 16 year old high school student experiencing debilitating anxiety for several months. She found it hard to sleep at night and couldn't concentrate in class. Her mother, concerned about her well-being, took her to a therapist specializing in Person-Centered Therapy.

Sophie had never been to therapy before and was apprehensive about sharing her innermost thoughts and feelings with a stranger.

The therapist began by asking Sophie to describe what had been happening in her life lately without judging or interpreting her experiences. Sophie hesitated initially but gradually opened up about her worries and fears. She talked about her difficulties with social anxiety and how she felt like she didn't fit in with her peers. She also shared that she was worried about her academic performance and felt like she was always falling behind.

The therapist listened carefully to Sophie's words and reflected on what she was hearing. "It sounds like you're feeling much pressure to fit in and do well in school," she said. "It's understandable that you're feeling anxious and overwhelmed."

Sophie nodded, grateful that someone was finally listening to her without trying to fix or judge her.

Over the next few weeks, Sophie continued to see the therapist and explore her feelings of anxiety. The therapist never told Sophie what to do or how to think but instead encouraged her to reflect on her experiences and find solutions. She would ask open-ended questions and offer gentle guidance when necessary, but she always allowed Sophie to take the lead in her therapy.

As Sophie gained more insight into her anxiety, she also developed a greater sense of self-acceptance and self-compassion. She realized that she didn't need to change who she was to fit in with her peers and that her academic performance did not determine her worth. With the therapist's support, she started challenging her negative self-talk and replacing it with more positive, self-affirming thoughts.

Eventually, Sophie's anxiety decreased and felt more confident and self-assured. She was able to sleep better at night and concentrate more in class. She even started making new friends and trying new things outside her comfort zone.

This is just one example of how the Person-Centered Approach can be used to treat teenage anxiety. By creating a safe and supportive environment where teenagers can explore their thoughts and feelings without fear of judgment or criticism, therapists can help them develop a greater sense of self-awareness and self-compassion.

This is how teenagers can develop a greater sense of personal well-being and manage their anxiety successfully.

It would help if you remember that a person enters person-centered therapy in incongruence. It is the role of the therapists to reverse this situation. Rogers (1959) called his therapeutic approach client-centered or person-centered therapy because of the focus on the person's subjective view of the world.

Congruenceis also called genuineness.Congruence is the most crucial attribute in counseling, according to Rogers. This means that, unlike the psychodynamic therapist, who generally maintains a passive stance and reveals little of their own personality in therapy, the humanistic therapist is keen to allow the client to experience them as they are.

Rogers espoused a philosophical tenet that everyone was an exclusive entity; hence, a one-size-fits-all approach would not meet everyone's needs (Kensit, 2000). Unlike some forms of psychotherapy, which consider a patient's thoughts, desires, and beliefs secondary to the therapeutic process, Rogers saw the client's experience as the most pivotal factor in the process.

Today, most of our current forms of therapy are rooted in the belief that the client is an equal partner in the therapeutic relationship rather than a powerless patient, and their experiences hold the key to personal growth and development as a singular individual.

Rogerian psychotherapy stands out from other therapies' fundamental belief that each individual can benefit from client-centered therapy and evolve from a "potentially competent individual" to a fully competent one (McLeod, 2015).

Rogers' approach perceives people as self-reliant individuals competent enough to undertake the effort required to realize their full potential and achieve positive life changes.

The general goals of the Person-Centered Approach are to:

Facilitate personal growth and development

Eliminate or mitigate feelings of distress

Increase self-esteem and openness to experience

Enhance the client's understanding of him- or herself Greater agreement between the client's idea and actual selves

Better understanding and awareness

Decreased defensiveness, insecurity, and guilt

Greater trust in oneself

Healthier relationships

Improvement in self-expression

Improved mental health overall

(Noel, 2018)

By looking at these goals, you can appreciate that the client (your teenager) is the expert in this form of therapy instead of the therapist.

Let us now delve into the merits and demerits of the Person-Centered Approach.

As discussed earlier, this approach emphasizes creating a safe, accepting, and empathic environment for clients to express their feelings, thoughts, and beliefs freely. The therapy is tailored to the client's needs, and the therapist takes a non-directive approach.

Pros of the Person-Centered Approach

1. Client Empowerment

The person-centered approach puts the client at the center of the therapeutic process. The therapist is a facilitator, creating a safe and supportive space where clients can explore their thoughts, feelings, and experiences. This approach empowers the client to take an active role in their own healing process, which can lead to more successful outcomes.

2. Non-Judgmental Environment

The person-centered approach is characterized by a non-judgmental, accepting, and empathetic stance on the therapist's part. The client is encouraged to explore their experiences without fear of being judged, which can help to create a more open and honest therapeutic relationship.

3. Flexibility

Person-centered therapy can be used to treat a wide range of mental health issues, including anxiety, depression, and relationship problems. This approach can be adapted to meet each client's unique needs, making it a flexible and versatile form of therapy.

4. Evidence-Based

Research has demonstrated the efficacy of person-centered therapy in the treatment of a variety of mental health issues.

A meta-analysis of 86 studies found that person-centered therapy was significantly more effective than no treatment or placebo treatment and was equally effective as other forms of psychotherapy (Elliott et al., 2011).

Cons of Person-Centered Approach

1. Lack of Direction

One of the criticisms of person-centered therapy is that it can lack direction or structure. Some clients may feel overwhelmed or unsure of where to begin when they are free to explore their experiences without guidance from the therapist.

2. Limited Effectiveness for Severe Mental Health Issues

While person-centered therapy can be effective for many mental health issues, it may not be the best approach for clients with severe mental health issues such as schizophrenia or bipolar disorder, in addition to anxiety. In these cases, more structured and directive forms of therapy may be necessary.

3. Potential for Dependency

Because person-centered therapy emphasizes the client's autonomy and self-direction, there is a risk that some clients may become overly reliant on the therapist for support and guidance. This can lead to a dependency that may hinder the client's progress.

4. Lack of Active Techniques

Person-centered therapy does not involve many active techniques, which some clients may find unhelpful. For example, clients who prefer more structured therapy may feel that person-centered therapy is too passive and unengaging.

Person-Centered Approach and Teen Anxiety

Person-centered therapy is a humanistic approach to psychotherapy that prioritizes the client's unique experience and individuality. It has gained popularity as a therapeutic approach to treating teen anxiety.

Person-centered therapy aims to provide clients with a supportive and non-judgmental environment to explore their inner selves and solve their problems. The therapist's role is to provide empathy, understanding, and unconditional positive regard toward the client, allowing them to feel validated, heard, and empowered to change their lives. The therapy focuses on the present and future rather than past events or traumas.

Several studies have explored the effectiveness of person-centered therapy for treating anxiety among teenagers. A randomized controlled trial by Levitt et al. (2006) found that person-centered therapy was more effective than cognitive-behavioral therapy in reducing anxiety symptoms among high school students.

Another study by McLeod and Jensen-Doss (2015) found that person-centered therapy was more effective than no therapy and as effective as other established treatments, including cognitive-behavioral therapy and psychodynamic therapy, in treating anxiety among young people.

Moreover, a study by Joffe and Zwerling (2004) suggests that person-centered therapy is particularly effective for anxious adolescents who have experienced early emotional trauma, such as abuse or neglect. The study found that clients who received person-centered therapy reported significant decreases in anxiety symptoms and improved self-esteem.

What to Look for in a Person-Centered Therapist?

No formal certification is required to practice person-centered therapy; licensed mental health professionals from various disciplines with training and experience in the approach can use it in therapy. In addition to finding someone with relevant background and experience, look for a therapist or counselor who is incredibly empathetic and with whom you feel comfortable discussing personal issues.

Therapists use the person-centered approach to form a robust therapeutic alliance with their clients. This helps maintain a stable and healthy relationship between the therapist and the client.

However, it is common for therapists to introduce and integrate various techniques from CBT, ACT, trauma-focused therapy, behavioral therapy, and modalities from other schools of thought according to the case and the client's need and pace.

Understanding that anxiety can manifest differently in people from different cultures and backgrounds is noteworthy. That's why embracing multiculturalism is so essential in helping our teens.

When we appreciate cultural diversity, we can understand the unique challenges that anxious teens face and create a personalized treatment plan that fits their needs.

For example, in some cultures, like the Asian culture, expressing emotions openly is not typical, so that anxiety may be shown through physical symptoms like stomach aches or headaches. It may also strongly emphasize collectivism, where anxiety may be linked to social obligations or family responsibilities.

It's also vital to acknowledge intersectionality, how different identities (like race, gender, or sexual orientation) intersect and affect a teen's anxiety.

When we target and address these issues, we can create a more holistic and effective treatment plan for our clients.

This proves that the person-centered approach is a foundation of therapy but is not limited or exclusive to it.

It is important to acknowledge that person-centered therapy benefits clients from diverse backgrounds to understand their issues and gain a deeper perspective of their troubles.

Conclusion

This approach allows the client to explore their thoughts and feelings, which can lead to increased self-awareness and personal growth. It also emphasizes the importance of empathy, genuineness, and positivity, which helps clients feel safe and comfortable in therapy.

Another advantage of the person-centered approach is its non-judgmental and non-critical stance. The therapist is not there to judge or criticize the client but to provide support and understanding. This lack of judgment and criticism can comfort clients, allowing them to be more open and honest about their feelings and experiences.

Additionally, the person-centered approach can help treat various mental health concerns, including anxiety, depression, and trauma. This therapy approach is often preferred by clients who have experienced negative therapy or are hesitant to try therapy due to fear of being judged or criticized.

However, there are also some potential drawbacks to the person-centered approach. One disadvantage is that it can be difficult for some clients to feel comfortable taking the therapy lead. Some clients may prefer a more directive approach and may feel overwhelmed by the open-ended nature of person-centered therapy.

Another potential disadvantage is that some clients may feel frustrated with the slow progress of therapy. This approach allows clients to set the pace, which can be slower than a more directive approach. Clients may feel impatient with the process and may need more structure and guidance to feel like they are making progress.

The person-centered approach can be challenging for therapists who are not comfortable with the non-directive nature of the therapy.

Some therapists may find it difficult to let go of control and allow the client to lead and may struggle to remain empathic and non-judgmental throughout the therapeutic process.

When trying to find a suitable therapist, it is crucial to self-reflect and decide what kind of therapy you are searching for. It takes time to fit a good fit, and you should not get discouraged if you don't find one after a few tries.

Each therapist has their own style and perspective of treating a client's issues. So, it is crucial that you visit a few whom you find to your liking and then decide on one who suits your personality best.

Most therapists offer a free initial consultation call that lasts for 15 minutes. Use this time to your advantage. Please don't shy away from asking your therapist about their approach to your issues during this initial consultation call.

It is common to start with person-centered therapy and switch to other modalities. Feel empowered to take the incentive and give input to your therapist about shifting to a different approach that suits your liking. This could be one or several more structured and directed techniques more aligned with your case. You will find that your therapist will be happily inclined to shift their style to meet your needs, goals, and pace.

Remember, person-centered therapy always puts the client first!

Overall, person-centered therapy can be a valuable treatment option for teenagers with anxiety, and several studies support its effectiveness.

We have come to the end of this chapter; I hope you have comprehended the person-centered therapeutic approach by now. I will leave you with a quote that encapsulates the true merit of self-empathy, a little food for thought, while we move on to the next treatment modality.

"He who knows others is wise; he who knows himself is enlightened."

-Lao Tzu

CHAPTER 6:

MINDFULNESS BOTTOM OF FORM

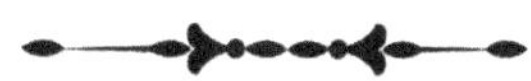

"People usually consider walking on water or in thin air a miracle. But I think the real miracle is not to walk either on water or in thin air, but to walk on earth. Every day we are engaged in a miracle which we don't even recognize: a blue sky, white clouds, green leaves, the black, curious eyes of a child—our own two eyes. All is a miracle." — **Thich Nhat Hanh, The Miracle of Mindfulness: An Introduction to the Practice of Meditation**

Welcome to the wonderful world of mindfulness, where the mundane becomes miraculous!

Thich Nhat Hanh's quote highlights the beauty and wonder of our daily lives and how often we take these simple joys for granted.

Mindfulness is being present and fully engaged in these everyday moments without judgments or distractions. It is a philosophy rooted in Buddhist teachings, but it has gained popularity and recognition in mainstream society for its potential to reduce stress and enhance overall well-being.

Mindfulness is about cultivating awareness and attention to the present moment. This involves training the mind to focus on the sensations, thoughts, and emotions that arise in each moment without getting swept away.

By developing this awareness, we can better understand our own patterns of thought and behavior and learn to respond to them with greater clarity and wisdom.

To practice mindfulness, one must first learn to be still and silent. It is all about absolving ourselves from our surroundings. This is not as easy as it may sound.

Why?

Our minds constantly race, jumping from one thought to the next, like a bullet train moving from one platform to another. But with practice, we can learn to slow down and focus on the present moment.

The most common technique for developing mindfulness is meditation. Meditation teaches us to observe our thoughts and emotions without getting caught up. We learn to cherry-pick the positive and discard the negative feelings. We become aware of the constant chatter in our minds and slowly learn to let go of our worries and fears.

Another way to practice mindfulness is to pay attention to our senses. This could be as simple as noticing the taste and texture of the food or the feeling of the sun on our skin. Being fully present at the moment allows us to experience even the most mundane activities with a sense of wonder and gratitude.

Non-judgment is a core principle of mindfulness. This means we approach our experiences with an open and curious attitude rather than labeling them as good or bad, right or wrong.

By letting go of these judgments, we can detach ourselves from the never-ending, vicious cycle of self-criticism and self-doubt that can damage our mental and emotional well-being.

Another essential aspect of mindfulness is acceptance. This means acknowledging and embracing our experiences, even the difficult or unpleasant ones, without trying to change or resist them. When we accept our experiences in this way, we can develop a sense of inner peace and resilience, even amid adverse circumstances.

The Origins of Mindfulness

Living mindfully involves being fully present and aware of the present moment rather than ruminating on the past or worrying about the future.

It entails objectively observing and labeling one's thoughts, emotions, and physical sensations. This approach can be a powerful tool for managing difficult emotions while avoiding self-judgment and criticism.

The roots of mindfulness can be traced back to ancient Hinduism and Buddhist teachings.

In Buddhism, the term *"sati"* encompasses concepts of attention, awareness, and presence and is seen as the first step toward enlightenment. The word "mindfulness" is a rough translation of this term from the ancient *Pali* language.

Introducing mindfulness into Western culture is primarily credited to Jon Kabat-Zinn, who studied under influential Buddhist teachers like Philip Kapleau and Thich Nhat Hanh.

In the late 1970s, Kabat-Zinn developed a program called Mindfulness-Based Stress Reduction (MBSR) to treat chronic pain. Through his research, he found that patients who practiced mindfulness were better able to manage their pain than those who attempted to avoid it.

Since then, mindfulness has become a fundamental technique in various therapeutic approaches such as Mindfulness-Based Cognitive Therapy, Dialectical Behavior Therapy, and Acceptance and Commitment Therapy.

Its widespread acceptance in the scientific and medical communities has led to its integration into mainstream society, making it a valuable tool for enhancing one's overall well-being.

The Advantages and Disadvantages of Mindfulness

Mindfulness has become a buzzword recently, with many people appreciating its benefits. While there are certainly advantages to practicing mindfulness, it's important also to consider its potential drawbacks.

Advantages of mindfulness:

1 Stress reduction

Mindfulness reduces stress by helping individuals become more aware of their thoughts and emotions. One can learn to manage stress more effectively by being present at the moment.

2. Improved focus

Mindfulness can help individuals improve their focus and concentration, as it requires paying attention to the present moment and tuning out distractions.

3. Increased self-awareness

Mindfulness can help individuals become more aware of their thoughts, emotions, and behaviors. This increased self-awareness can lead to personal growth and self-improvement.

4. Better relationships

Mindfulness can help individuals become more empathetic and compassionate towards others. This can lead to improved relationships and better communication.

5. Improved physical health

Mindfulness has been shown to have physical health benefits, such as reducing blood pressure and improving sleep quality.

Disadvantages of mindfulness:

1. Time commitment

Practicing mindfulness requires time and effort. It may be challenging for some individuals to find the time to practice mindfulness regularly.

2. Initial discomfort

When starting a mindfulness practice, some individuals may experience discomfort or unease as they become more aware of their thoughts and emotions.

3. Potential for emotional overload

Mindfulness can bring up difficult emotions, and some individuals may find it overwhelming to confront them.

4. Overemphasis on individual responsibility

Mindfulness can sometimes be promoted as a solution to individual problems, which can overlook social, economic, and political factors' role in shaping our experiences.

5. Not a panacea/ one-size-fits-all approach

While mindfulness can help manage stress and improve well-being, it is not a cure-all for mental health problems. Individuals with serious mental health conditions should seek professional help.

We must remember that mindfulness can be a valuable tool for improving well-being and relationships. However, it's important to approach it critically and understand that it may not fit everyone.

Common Misconceptions About Mindfulness

We often wonder, is mindfulness the same as flow state?

Well, no. Mindfulness and flow state are two distinct concepts.

Mindfulness is the practice of being present and non-judgmentally aware of your thoughts, feelings, and surroundings in the present moment.

It involves intentionally bringing your focus to the present and observing your experiences without getting caught up in or reacting to them. Mindfulness can be practiced through meditation, but it can also be incorporated into daily activities.

Flow state, on the other hand, is a mental state of complete absorption and focus in an activity. When in a flow state, you are fully immersed in the present moment and lose track of time and any sense of self-consciousness or external distractions.

Flow state is often experienced during activities that require a high level of skill and challenge, such as sports, music, or creative endeavors.

While both mindfulness and flow state involve being present in the moment, mindfulness is a deliberate practice that can be applied to any situation, while flow state is a state of mind that occurs spontaneously during certain activities. Additionally, mindfulness involves observing and accepting whatever arises in the present moment, while the flow state consists in being fully absorbed and focused on the task at hand.

So, are mindfulness and meditation interchangeable?

Again, no. Mindfulness and meditation are related concepts, but they are not interchangeable.

Mindfulness is a mental state characterized by present-moment awareness and non-judgmental acceptance of one's thoughts, emotions, and bodily sensations.

Meditation, on the other hand, is a specific practice or technique that is frequently used to cultivate mindfulness. Meditation involves intentionally focusing on a particular object, such as the breath, a sound, or a mantra, to quiet the mind and develop a sense of inner calm and clarity.

While mindfulness can be practiced informally throughout the day by paying attention to the present moment, meditation is usually done in a formal, seated position. It involves setting aside a specific amount of time to focus on cultivating a particular state of mind.

Mindfulness in Action

Engaging a teenager in mindfulness practices can be challenging, but it can be done with a little creativity and flexibility.

One of the most effective ways to encourage a teenager to practice mindfulness is to make it a fun and engaging activity. Here are some ways to do that:

1. Mindful activities

Engage your teenager in mindful activities that they enjoy. For example, if your teenager likes to draw, encourage them to create a mindful drawing to focus on the present moment and their feelings. Other examples of mindful activities could be walking, yoga, art or music therapy, cooking or gardening. These activities can help teenagers connect with their bodies and develop greater awareness of their thoughts and emotions.

2. Technology

Teenagers love technology, so why not use it to engage them in mindfulness?

Several mindfulness apps are available that can be easily downloaded and used on smartphones or tablets. These apps offer guided meditations, breathing exercises, and other mindfulness practices that can be done anywhere and anytime.

3. Social support

Encourage your teenager to practice mindfulness with friends. This can be done through a mindfulness group or a simple activity like mindful coloring or yoga. Peer support can be a powerful motivator for teenagers.

4. Role modeling

As a parent or caregiver, you can model mindfulness practices yourself. If your teenager sees you practicing mindfulness regularly, they are more likely to adopt it themselves.

5. Incorporate into the daily routine.

Encourage your teenager to incorporate mindfulness into their daily routine. This can be done by setting aside a few minutes daily for meditation or mindful breathing.

Mindfulness scripts

Mindfulness scripts are pre-written guided meditations that are used to lead individuals through mindfulness practice. These scripts can be helpful for beginners who are just starting to explore mindfulness or for those who struggle to focus during their training. Mindfulness scripts can also be a powerful tool for engaging teenagers in mindful practices.

They can help walk teenagers through becoming more present and aware. They can be used in various settings, such as classrooms, therapy sessions, or at home. A teacher can read the scripts aloud or record them for personal use.

There are many different types of mindfulness scripts, each with its focus and intention. Some scripts focus on body awareness, while others focus on breath awareness or visualization techniques. Many scripts also incorporate elements of self-compassion and gratitude.

To use a mindfulness script, the teenager should find a quiet, comfortable place to sit or lie down. The script should be read slowly and in a calming tone, guiding the teenager through exercises such as deep breathing, body scans, and visualization.

Giving the teenager time to process each exercise before moving on to the next one is essential. It can also be helpful to set an intention for the practice beforehand, such as reducing stress or increasing self-awareness.

Once you have found a quiet space and set your intention, start by reading or playing the mindfulness script. Follow along with the instructions, focusing on the breath or other sensations as directed.

If your mind wanders, acknowledge the thought and gently bring your attention back to the present moment.

An example of a mindfulness script for teenagers is a body scan meditation. In this meditation, the teenager is guided to focus on each part of their body, starting from their toes and working their way up to their head. They are asked to notice any sensations or feelings in each body part without judgment or analysis.

The advantage of mindfulness scripts is that they can provide structure and guidance for those new to the practice. They can also be helpful for those who struggle with racing thoughts or distractions during their practice. Additionally, mindfulness scripts can be adapted to meet the needs of individuals with different experience levels or specific needs, such as those with anxiety or depression.

However, it is vital to note that mindfulness scripts are not a one-size-fits-all solution. Some individuals may find them too structured or may have difficulty following along with the instructions. Listening to your body and adapting the practice as needed is central.

Some teenagers may find it difficult or uncomfortable to practice mindfulness. It is important to respect their feelings and not force them to participate. It's essential to allow teenagers to find their path and engage in practices that work for them.

Walking Meditation Guided Script

For this meditation, find a quiet place indoors with space to walk in small circles, or choose a path or quiet open space outdoors.

We'll begin standing. Close your eyes with your feet at hips width apart, and your arms hang loose by your sides.

Wherever you are, root your feet to the ground, and feel the opposing energy that transfers from the earth up through your spine and the crown of your head.

Notice how the more you press down into the earth, the taller you feel.

Let breath awareness guide your attention toward your body. Focus on the connection between your feet and the ground, and sensation in your legs and low body.

Spend a few cycles of breath here, simply noticing what is. Where the body is. How does the body feel?

With your eyes still closed, slowly shift back and forth from your heels to the balls of your feet a few times.

Notice what arises in your awareness with this slight movement. Then return to neutral and get centered.

And shift side to side—just a tiny sway of your weight from the right foot to the left, back and forth.

Or from the outer edge of the foot towards the inner arches. Notice what arises in your awareness with this small movement.

Return to the center, and focus your energy again on noticing the connection between your feet and the earth.

The sensations of your lower body, thighs, knees, calves, shins, heels, inner arches and ankles, the soles of your feet and toes. Maintain this awareness of your felt sense of the body as you slowly open your eyes.

Still standing for a few cycles of breath as you take in the information of the body, in spite of the distractions of all that you see.

As you are ready, with body awareness, begin slowly walking forward.

Take as much time as you can with each movement and each part of every movement.

Notice all the detail you can. The shift of your weight forward. The shift from the heel toward the toes The lift of the heel The lift of the foot

(https://mindfulnessexercises.com/walking-meditation-guided-script/)

A Mindful Eating Script

Connect to your breath and body, feel your feet on the ground, and notice your experience. With your awareness, notice any thoughts, sensations, or emotions you are experiencing. (Pause)

Tune into the awareness or sensation you have in your body of feeling hungry, thirsty or maybe even full. If you were going to eat or drink something right now, what is your body hungry for? What is it thirsty for? Pay attention and notice with awareness the sensations that give you this information. (Pause)

Now, bring your attention to the item in your hand and imagine seeing it for the first time. Observe with curiosity as you pay attention and notice the color, shape, texture, and size. Is there anything else that you see, sense, or feel? (Pause)

Imagine what it took for this item to get to your hands: sunshine, water, time, processing, and shipping. You may choose to be aware of gratitude for everyone involved in the cultivation and preparation of this item of food. You may choose to bring in your own appreciation or spiritual blessing. (Pause)

Now place the item between your fingers and feel the texture, temperature, and ridges. You may notice smoothness or stickiness. Again, see your thoughts, sensations, or emotions now. Continue to breathe and be fully present in this moment. (Pause)

Take the piece of food and bring it toward your nose and smell with your full awareness. Notice if you have any memories, sensations, or reactions in your body. Even before you eat it, you may notice that you begin to have a digestive response just by seeing and smelling it. (Pause)

With full awareness of your hand moving toward your mouth, place the object (fruit or chocolate) into your mouth without chewing or swallowing it. Just allow it to be in your mouth, and roll it around to different parts of your mouth and tongue.

Notice the flavor and texture. Notice the physical sensations within your body, especially your mouth and gut. Continue to breathe as you explore the feeling of having this item in your mouth. (Pause)

Next, take just one bite and notice the flavor and change of texture. Then very slowly, begin to chew this piece of food, and notice the parts of your mouth involved in chewing. Notice the sound and movement of chewing as you continue to witness the sensations and flavor. (Pause)

When you are ready, swallow this item and notice its path from your mouth and throat into your stomach. Notice the sensation and taste that may linger in your mouth.

Connect again to your body and your breath, and notice your experience. (Pause)

Next, I invite you to pick up another food item and choose to eat it however you wish. You are noticing your choice and your experience. Notice how it is similar or different. (Pause for 30-60 seconds, then return to an extensive group discussion about the experience).

(The Mindful Eating Script written by Christine MilovaniLCSW, based on information from KabatZinn's book Full Catastrophe Living: Using the Wisdom of Your Body and Mind to Face Stress, Pain, and Illness published by Delacorte Press in 2013 and McWatter's article Mindful Eating 101: Eating in the Present Moment)

A Mindful Breathing Script

Start by settling into a comfortable position and allow your eyes to close or keep them open with a softened gaze.

Begin by taking several long slow deep breaths breathing in fully and exhaling fully.

Breathe in through your nose and out through your nose or mouth.

Allow your breath to find its natural rhythm. Bring your attention to noticing each in-breath as it enters your nostrils, travels down to your lungs, and causes your belly to expand. And notice each out-breath as your belly contracts and air moves up through the lungs back up through the nostrils or mouth.

Invite your full attention to flow with your breath. Notice how the inhale is different from the exhale. You may experience the air as cool as it enters your nose and warm as you exhale.

As you turn more deeply inward, begin to let go of noises around you. If you are distracted by sounds in the room, notice them and bring your intention back to your breath. Breathe as you breathe, not striving to change anything about your breath. Don't try to control your breath in any way.

Observe and accept your experience without judgment, paying attention to each inhale and exhale. If your mind wanders to thoughts, plans, or problems, just notice your mind wandering.

Watch the thought as it enters your awareness as neutrally as possible. Then practice letting go of the thought like a leaf floating down a stream. In your mind, place each thought that arises on a leaf and watch as it flows out of sight down the stream.

Then bring your attention back to your breath. Your breath is an anchor you can return to over and over again when you become distracted by thoughts. Notice when your mind has wandered.

Observe the types of thoughts that hook or distract you. Noticing is the wealthiest part of learning. With this knowledge, you can strengthen your ability to detach from thoughts and mindfully focus your awareness back on the qualities of your breath.

Practice coming home to the breath with your full attention. Watching the gentle rise of your stomach on the in-breath and the relaxing, letting go on the out-breath.

Allow yourself to be complete with your breath as it flows in and out. You might become distracted by pain or discomfort in the body or twitching or itching sensations that draw your attention away from the breath. You may also notice feelings arising, perhaps sadness or happiness, frustration or contentment.

Acknowledge whatever comes up, including thoughts or stories about your experience. Notice where your mind went without judging it, pushing it away, clinging to it, or wishing it were different, and simply refocus your mind and guide your attention back to your breath.

Breathe in and out. Follow the air all the way in and all the way out. Mindfully, be present moment by moment with your breath. If your mind wanders away from your breath, just notice without judging it – be it a thought, emotion, or sensation that hooks your attention and gently guides your awareness back to your breathing.

As this practice ends, slowly allow your attention to expand and notice your entire body and then beyond your body to the room you are in.

When you're ready, open your eyes and come back fully alert and awake.

The breath is always with you as a refocusing tool to bring you back to the present moment. Set your intention to use this practice throughout your day to help cultivate and strengthen attention.

(Script written by Shilagh Mirgain, Ph.D., for UW Cultivating Well-Being: A Neuroscientific Approach)

Benefits of Mindfulness

Mindfulness has been widely studied and has been found to have a range of benefits for both physical and mental health.

One of the main benefits of mindfulness is *stress reduction*. Studies have shown that mindfulness can reduce stress and anxiety levels, lower blood pressure, and improve overall cardiovascular health (Khoury et al., 2015; Pascoe et al., 2017).

Another benefit of mindfulness is its ability to improve *cognitive functioning*, including attention, memory, and decision-making (Zeidan et al., 2010). Regular mindfulness practice has been shown to increase grey matter in areas of the brain associated with attention and emotion regulation (Hölzel et al., 2011).

Mindfulness has also been effective in treating various mental health conditions, including depression, anxiety disorders, and substance abuse (Goldberg et al., 2018; Garland et al., 2015; Bowen et al., 2014). Mindfulness-based interventions have been shown to reduce symptoms of depression and anxiety and improve emotional regulation and overall well-being (Segal et al., 2010).

Mindfulness has also been linked to *improved sleep quality* (Black et al., 2015), *increased immune functioning* (Davidson et al., 2003), and even *improved relationships* (Carson et al., 2004).

Mindfulness-based interventions are effective in reducing symptoms of depression and anxiety and improving emotional regulation and overall well-being.

Mindfulness and Teenage Anxiety

Mindfulness has been proven to be an effective tool in managing anxiety in teenagers. Anxiety is a common mental health problem among teenagers, and it can negatively influence their daily lives, including academic performance and social interactions. Mindfulness interventions aim to increase awareness and acceptance of present-moment experiences without judgment and can be adapted for use in various settings such as schools, clinics, and homes.

Several studies have investigated the effectiveness of mindfulness in reducing anxiety among teenagers. One study found that an eight-week mindfulness-based stress reduction (MBSR) program significantly reduced adolescent anxiety symptoms. The study involved 102 adolescents randomly assigned to an eight-week mindfulness program or a control group. The mindfulness program included group sessions and home practice and focused on mindfulness techniques such as body scans, breathing exercises, and meditation. The results showed that the mindfulness group significantly reduced anxiety and depression symptoms compared to the control group, and these improvements were maintained at a six-month follow-up (Biegel et al., 2009).

Another study found that a mindfulness-based intervention reduced anxiety symptoms and improved emotional regulation among adolescents with anxiety disorders (Semple et al., 2010).

By practicing mindfulness, teenagers can learn to observe and label their thoughts and emotions objectively, rather than getting caught up in them. This can help them to develop a sense of control and mastery over their feelings, reducing the sense of helplessness that often accompanies anxiety.

Mindfulness has also been found to positively impact the brain, specifically in areas related to emotional regulation and stress response. Research has shown that mindfulness can increase activity in the prefrontal cortex, the part of the brain responsible for executive function and decision-making, and decrease activity in the amygdala, which is responsible for the stress response (Tang et al., 2015).

Another study published in the Journal of Adolescence examined the effectiveness of a school-based mindfulness program for reducing anxiety symptoms and improving academic performance in a group of high school students (Weare & Nind, 2011). The said program involves weekly mindfulness sessions, home practice, and integration of mindfulness practices into daily routines. The results showed that the mindfulness program effectively reduced anxiety symptoms, improved academic performance, and increased mindfulness and self-compassion.

A meta-analysis published in the Journal of Child and Family Studies found that mindfulness-based interventions effectively reduced anxiety symptoms in children and adolescents (Burke, Langer, & Germer, 2010). The meta-analysis included 10 studies with a total of 226 participants and found that mindfulness interventions led to significant reductions in anxiety symptoms. The researchers noted that mindfulness-based interventions may be particularly effective for individuals with higher levels of anxiety or those with a history of anxiety disorders.

Therefore, mindfulness can be an effective tool for teenagers struggling with anxiety. It can help them develop greater emotional regulation and resilience, improving overall well-being.

Well, we've come to the end of our mindfulness journey!

After discussing the concept and philosophy of mindfulness, the various ways to engage teenagers in mindfulness practices, and the benefits of mindfulness, it's safe to say that mindfulness is a powerful concept that can be used for living a more peaceful, fulfilling life.

Whether you're a teenager struggling with anxiety or an adult seeking a way to manage stress, incorporating mindfulness practices into your daily routine can profoundly affect your mental and physical well-being.

There are plenty of ways to practice mindfulness, from meditation to mindful breathing and body scans. And don't worry. You don't have to be a master meditator to reap the benefits. Being present in the moment and observing your thoughts and feelings with non-judgmental awareness can make a world of difference.

So, take a deep breath, let go of any expectations, and try mindfulness. Who knows, you might find yourself walking on the sunshine!

CHAPTER 7:

INTERPERSONAL PSYCHOTHERAPY

"You may not control all the events that happen to you, but you can decide not to be reduced by them."

— Maya Angelou

Being a psychologist, I aspire to help individuals struggling with anxiety and other mental health challenges find relief and lead happier and well-balanced lives.

Psychotherapy has shown, time and again, its boundless returns in the field of psychology.

Let's examine how psychotherapy can be an invaluable tool for managing your teen's anxiety.

Psychotherapy is a talk therapy involving working with a trained mental health professional to explore and address psychological and emotional difficulties.

Psychotherapy aims to help individuals gain insight into their thoughts, feelings, and behaviors and develop coping strategies to manage and overcome their challenges.

Interpersonal psychotherapy (IPT) is a specific type of psychotherapy that focuses on interpersonal relationships and social functioning. IPT is based on the idea that social relationships and life events can contribute to developing and maintaining mental health problems, including anxiety.

In IPT, the therapist works with the individual to identify and address problems in their interpersonal relationships, such as communication difficulties, conflicts, and social isolation. The therapist helps the individual learn new communication and problem-solving skills and develop healthier, more rewarding relationships.

IPT can be especially helpful for anxious teenagers struggling with social anxiety and difficulty making and maintaining relationships. When teenagers work with their therapist, they can learn to communicate better with their peers, develop more vital social skills, and manage their anxiety in social situations.

I have seen firsthand the benefits of IPT for parents and anxious teenagers. IPT can help parents and teenagers learn how to communicate more effectively, address conflicts in a healthy manner, and develop a stronger bond. It can also help teenagers build self-esteem and improve their overall social functioning.

IPT VS Other Treatment Modalities

Interpersonal therapy was developed in the 1970s by Gerald Klerman and Myrna Weissman. IPT has been shown to be an effective treatment for various mental health disorders, including depression, anxiety, and eating disorders.

The principle of IPT is based on the idea that interpersonal problems and conflicts can trigger and exacerbate mental health issues. IPT addresses these problems and helps individuals to develop more effective communication and problem-solving skills. It aims to improve their psychological well-being.

IPT is a time-limited therapy that typically lasts between 12 and 16 sessions, focusing on identifying and addressing specific interpersonal problems within this time frame.

Compared to other treatment modalities, IPT has some unique features. The pivotal notion of IPT is that it is highly focused on the patient's interpersonal difficulties. Unlike different approaches, such as cognitive-behavioral therapy, which may focus on thoughts and behaviors, IPT is targeted at helping patients identify and resolve interpersonal issues that are causing distress.

This approach may be particularly beneficial for individuals experiencing relationship difficulties and may benefit from learning more effective communication skills.

IPT has been shown to be effective in treating depression, with some studies indicating that it is as effective as cognitive-behavioral therapy (CBT) and other forms of psychotherapy (Cuijpers et al., 2016; Cuijpers et al., 2013).

IPT has also been effective in treating anxiety disorders (Markowitz et al., 2015) and eating disorders (Fairburn et al., 2015). One study found that IPT was more effective than the treatment as usual for patients with social anxiety disorder (Kaplan et al., 2015).

Compared to medication-based treatments, IPT is as effective in treating depression and anxiety (Cuijpers et al., 2013; Markowitz et al., 2015) and may be a more acceptable option for some patients who prefer non-pharmacological approaches. IPT may have longer-lasting effects than medication-based treatments, as it addresses underlying interpersonal issues that may contribute to developing mental health conditions.

How Does Interpersonal Therapy Work?

To understand this, we must first acknowledge the different types of Interpersonal therapy.

Interpersonal psychotherapy for depression (IPT-D)

This type of therapy is specifically designed to treat depression by addressing issues related to interpersonal relationships, such as communication difficulties, conflicts, and losses. It typically is structured around four phases: assessment, identification of problem areas, intervention, and termination. The therapist helps the patient to identify specific areas of difficulty in their relationships and to develop strategies for improving them.

Interpersonal psychotherapy for adolescents (IPT-A)

This type of therapy is similar to IPT-D, but it is tailored specifically to the needs of teenagers. It is designed to help adolescents develop better communication and problem-solving skills and cope with common issues such as conflicts with parents and peers, school problems, and romantic relationships.

Brief interpersonal psychotherapy (BIPT)

This is a shorter and more focused version of IPT. It typically involves 6-8 weekly sessions and is designed to address a specific problem area, such as grief, conflict resolution, or life transitions.

Cognitive Interpersonal Therapy (CIT)

This focuses on helping individuals change negative patterns of thinking and behavior that contribute to interpersonal problems. The therapy also seeks to improve communication skills, increase self-awareness, and help individuals develop coping mechanisms for dealing with difficult interpersonal situations. CIT often treats depression, anxiety, and other mental health disorders.

Dynamic Interpersonal Therapy (DIT)

This form of psychodynamic therapy emphasizes the importance of interpersonal relationships and how they affect our mental and emotional well-being. DIT aims to help individuals better understand their thoughts and feelings, as well as the thoughts and feelings of others. The therapy typically consists of 16 sessions over a period of five months.

Interpersonal and Social Rhythm Therapy (IPSRT)

Interpersonal and social rhythm therapy (IPSRT) is a type of psychotherapy that is often used to treat bipolar disorder. IPSRT combines elements of interpersonal therapy and cognitive-behavioral therapy, focusing on regulating daily routines and maintaining regular social rhythms. The therapy helps individuals develop healthy sleep patterns, regular meal schedules, and consistent exercise habits and improve their communication and problem-solving skills in their interpersonal relationships.

Metacognitive Interpersonal Therapy (MIT)

This integrative approach to treating personality disorders involves emotional inhibition or avoidance. MIT focuses on developing metacognitive awareness, which refers to observing and understanding one's thoughts and emotions. The therapy also helps individuals improve their interpersonal relationships by teaching them how to regulate their emotions better and respond to the feelings of others. MIT typically involves 12 weeks of therapy sessions.

An IP therapist assists the client in understanding how their interpersonal interactions and relationships may impact their emotional and mental health. To achieve this, the therapist will implement a set of techniques. They are as follows.

Interpersonal Inventory

In this technique, the therapist and the client work together to identify the client's essential relationships and any problems or conflicts that may be present in those relationships. The therapist helps the client explore how these problems may impact the client's emotional and mental health and identify specific goals for addressing the issues.

Role Playing

In this technique, the therapist helps the client to practice new ways of interacting with others. For example, if the client struggles with assertiveness in their relationships, the therapist may role-play a situation with the client in which they practice expressing their needs and setting boundaries. Role-playing can help clients build their confidence and develop new interpersonal skills.

Communication Analysis

In this technique, the therapist and client work together to analyze specific communication patterns that may be causing problems in the client's relationships. For example, if the client is struggling with conflict in their relationship with their parent, the therapist may help them identify communication patterns that contribute to the competition, such as negative language or poor listening skills. The client can learn to communicate more effectively and reduce conflict by identifying these patterns.

Problem-Solving

In this technique, the therapist and client work together to identify problems that are causing distress in the client's life and develop strategies for addressing those problems. This may involve identifying resources the client can use to address the issue, such as social support or practical help, or developing specific action plans to address the problem.

Grief Work

In this technique, the therapist helps the client process and cope with losing a loved one. This may involve exploring the client's feelings about the loss, working through any unfinished business or unresolved conflicts related to the loss, and developing strategies for coping with the grief.

Let's explore IPT in action with a story of a fictional teenager named Sarah.

Sarah was a 16-year-old high school student who was struggling with feelings of anxiety and depression. She found it difficult to make friends, often felt isolated, and had a strained relationship with her parents.

During the initial sessions, Sarah worked with her therapist to identify the interpersonal problems contributing to her mental health issues.

The therapist used countless techniques to explore Sarah's thoughts and feelings, including open-ended questions, active listening, and empathy.

One of the first areas that Sarah and her therapist explored was her difficulty making friends. The therapist used the technique of role-playing to help Sarah develop her social skills and build her confidence. Through these sessions, Sarah became more aware of her body language and tone of voice when speaking to others and learned to communicate her thoughts and feelings more effectively.

As Sarah continued with therapy, she began recognizing the patterns in her relationships with her parents. She often felt that they were overly critical and didn't understand her. The therapist helped Sarah express her feelings to her parents safely and constructively and

Throughout the course of therapy, Sarah's relationships with her peers and family began to improve. She reported feeling less anxious and more confident in communicating with others. The skills she learned in therapy also helped her navigate future interpersonal challenges.

Interpersonal Therapy and Emotional Intelligence

Interpersonal therapy (IPT) and emotional intelligence (EI) are interrelated concepts in many ways. Emotional intelligence is the ability to recognize, understand, and regulate one's own emotions as well as the emotions of others. Interpersonal therapy, on the other hand, is a type of talk therapy that focuses on improving relationships and interpersonal functioning.

The central theme of interpersonal therapy is to help individuals improve their ability to communicate and connect with others healthily and effectively. To do this, IPT often involves a focus on emotional expression and regulation. Clients are encouraged to explore their feelings and express them in a clear and constructive way while also learning how to manage difficult emotions and navigate challenging interpersonal situations.

In this sense, emotional intelligence plays a critical role in the success of interpersonal therapy. When they develop greater emotional awareness and regulation skills, individuals are better equipped to understand and express their own emotions and interpret and respond to the feelings of others. This can help facilitate more effective communication, reduce interpersonal conflict, and improve overall well-being.

Interpersonal therapy can also help to develop emotional intelligence by promoting greater empathy and understanding of others. Through exploring and processing past interpersonal experiences, individuals can better understand how their behavior and emotions impact those around them.

This can contribute to greater empathy and emotional intelligence as individuals learn to recognize and respond to the emotional needs of others more effectively and compassionately.

Interpersonal Therapy Exercises

Therapists use various exercises in IPT to help their clients improve their relationships with others, regulate their emotions, and manage stress.

Guided Imagery and Re-scripting

With this exercise, the client imagines themselves in a traumatic or upsetting situation and then visualizes how they would handle it more effectively. The goal is to help the client desensitize to their fears and anxieties and learn new, positive coping methods.

Drama Technique

This is another approach used in IPT, which involves role-playing problematic scenarios and exploring how different actions and words can lead to different outcomes. Through drama therapy, clients can practice new behaviors and build empathy, which can help them develop deeper insights and understand other people's perspectives.

Bodily Work

This is another technique used in IPT. This involves exercises such as grounding, breath regulation, and physical training to help clients regulate their emotions and improve their physical and mental well-being. Through experiencing strong physical states, clients can break damaging interpersonal patterns and learn to access positive self-images.

Mindfulness and Attention Regulation

These are also essential exercises in IPT. These techniques help clients become self-aware, recognize that thoughts are not facts, and develop a sense of agency. Clients can reduce stress, improve their emotional regulation, and increase their awareness by paying attention to their body's internal signals, position in a room, and sounds.

The Mood Thermometer

This visual guide is used in IPT to help clients track their moods and identify the associated interpersonal interactions. This exercise is beneficial for children struggling to identify and express their emotions.

The Closeness Circle

This is another visual guide that helps clients identify patterns of difficulty in maintaining strong interpersonal relationships. By focusing on interpersonal skills, clients can better understand their meaningful relationships and develop strategies for improving them.

Worksheets are also used in IPT to help clients explore and understand their relationships with others.

The Interpersonal Relationships worksheet prompts clients to describe their relationships, what they like and dislike about the person, and how the relationship impacts them.

The Interpersonal Parenting Tips worksheet provides practical tips for parents to strengthen their relationship with their children, while **the Wanting to Be Heard** worksheet gives clients valuable information for effective communication.

Emotional Repetition and Attention Remodeling

These techniques help clients desensitize negative feelings that arise under challenging situations. By identifying common negative phrases and practicing attention remodeling, clients can decrease or eliminate negative emotions and build emotional resilience.

The Benefits of Interpersonal Psychotherapy

The most remarkable advantage of IPT is that it is a time-limited therapy. This means that clients can achieve meaningful results relatively quickly, which is particularly helpful for those who may not have the time or resources to commit to longer-term therapy.

It's a structured, formulaic approach that makes it easier to track progress. It also has the flexibility to extend into long-term therapy for those individuals who prefer and have complex challenges.

Another noteworthy benefit of IPT is that it is evidence-based, meaning that it has been extensively researched and shown to be effective for a range of mental health concerns, including depression, anxiety, and eating disorders. Research has consistently demonstrated that IPT can significantly improve symptoms, quality of life, and overall functioning.

A significant advantage of IPT is that it is a focused therapy that explicitly targets interpersonal issues, such as communication difficulties, relationship conflicts, and social isolation. By addressing these issues directly, IPT can help clients to develop the skills and strategies they need to improve their relationships and enhance their social support networks. This, in turn, can lead to improved mood and greater emotional resilience.

IPT is also a collaborative and supportive form of therapy, which can be particularly beneficial for clients struggling with feelings of loneliness, isolation, or disconnection. The therapist works closely with the client to identify their goals and develop a treatment plan tailored to their needs. This collaborative approach helps to build trust and rapport between the therapist and client, which can be a significant factor in the success of the therapy.

Another benefit of IPT is that it is a flexible therapy that can be adapted to suit the needs of different clients. The therapist can use various techniques and exercises to help the client achieve their goals, including guided imagery, role-playing, and mindfulness-based exercises. By drawing on a range of different approaches, the therapist can create a treatment plan tailored to the client's specific needs and preferences.

IPT is a strengths-based therapy focusing on building on the client's strengths and resources. Rather than focusing solely on the client's weaknesses or problems, IPT encourages them to identify their existing skills and abilities and use these to overcome their interpersonal difficulties. This positive and empowering approach can help clients feel more confident and capable, which can substantially impact their overall well-being and mental health.

The Efficacy of Interpersonal Psychotherapy

Interpersonal psychotherapy (IPT) has shown promising results in treating teenage anxiety and other mental illnesses.

In a randomized controlled trial of IPT for adolescents with major depressive disorder, it was found to be effective in reducing symptoms and improving functioning (Young et al., 2016).

IPT has also been shown to be effective in treating anxiety disorders in adolescents, including generalized anxiety disorder and social anxiety disorder (Hofmann and Smits, 2017).

One study compared the efficacy of IPT to cognitive-behavioral therapy (CBT) in treating adolescent depression and found that both treatments were equally effective in reducing depressive symptoms (Mufson et al., 2010). However, another study found that IPT was more effective than CBT in reducing depressive symptoms in adolescents with comorbid anxiety disorders (Lipschitz et al., 2019).

Apart from anxiety and depression, IPT has also been studied in treating other mental illnesses in adolescents. In a randomized controlled trial, IPT effectively reduced symptoms of post-traumatic stress disorder (PTSD) in adolescents who had experienced a single incident of trauma (Cohen et al., 2017). IPT has also shown promise in treating eating disorders in adolescents, with one study finding it to be effective in reducing symptoms of binge eating disorder (Wilfley et al., 2010).

Like any treatment modality, Interpersonal psychotherapy has its limitations.

IPT may not be suitable for individuals with severe or chronic mental illnesses requiring more intensive interventions, such as medication management or hospitalization. In such cases, IPT may be used with other treatments, but it may not be sufficient as a standalone treatment.

IPT also may not be effective for all individuals. While studies have shown that IPT can be effective for some individuals with anxiety and other mental illnesses, not all may respond to this type of therapy. Some clients may require a different kind of therapy or a combination of therapies to manage their symptoms effectively.

IPT may not be accessible to all individuals, particularly those in underserved or marginalized communities. Barriers to access, such as cost, transportation, and stigma, may prevent some individuals from seeking or receiving IPT.

One potential weakness of IPT is its shorter timeline, which may not offer enough support for people with chronic or relapsing mental health issues. IPT practitioners recognize that maintenance sessions may be necessary for recurring symptoms.

Also, its formulaic approach may mean that therapy does not offer relief if a person drops out early or cannot pay for continued treatment.

IPT requires a high level of training and expertise on the therapist's part. Not all therapists may have the necessary training or experience to implement IPT effectively. This may limit the availability of IPT as a treatment option for some individuals.

Despite these limitations, IPT remains a valuable treatment option for many individuals with anxiety and other mental illnesses.

How to Approach Your Therapist For IPT

If you're considering seeking Interpersonal Psychotherapy (IPT) for your teenager, knowing what to expect and how to find the right therapist is essential.

Your therapist will begin by learning more about your teen, their symptoms, and their relationship history. Then, your teen and the therapist will work together to identify and address specific problem areas. The therapist will adapt strategies and approaches based on your teen's progress throughout treatment.

A good therapist should also help your teen identify any interpersonal issues they want to address, offer support for communication analysis and clarification of problems, and provide supportive listening throughout their treatment.

To find an IPT therapist, you can look in clinics, private practices, or other mental health institutions. Screening potential therapists to ensure they have experience treating your concerns is important.

During the initial consultation, you can ask the therapist questions such as how they plan to address your specific concerns, whether they have dealt with similar problems before and the process and timeline for treatment.

Your doctor can also help you determine if IPT fits your teen's needs and whether it would be more effective if combined with other treatments.

It's important to remember that finding the right therapist and treatment approach can take time, but with the proper support, your teen can make positive changes in their mental health.

Well, we've come to the end of our chapter on interpersonal psychotherapy, and what a journey it's been!

From learning about the history and development of IPT to exploring its efficacy in treating various mental illnesses, we've covered much ground.

We've discussed about's benefits of IPT, including improved communication, better relationships, and reduced symptoms of depression and anxiety.

We've also discussed some limitations, like its focus on interpersonal issues and potential difficulty addressing deeper, underlying psychological issues.

It's safe to say that interpersonal psychotherapy is a superlative treatment option for those struggling with mental health issues, especially those related to relationships and social interactions. It's important to find a therapist trained in IPT and can provide a structured, supportive environment for treatment.

I hope this brief overview has piqued your interest and inspired you to seek more information and resources on your own.

And hey, if all else fails, maybe just try being a good listener and communicator to your teen - that might be the best therapy!

CHAPTER 8:

ACCEPTANCE AND COMMITMENT THERAPY

Let's explore Acceptance and Commitment Therapy (ACT), a type of psychotherapy that focuses on accepting what is out of our control and committing to actions that enrich our lives.

Robert Greene, in his book, "48 Laws of Power" aptly puts,

"Accept that all events occur for a reason and that it is within your capacity to see this reason as positive."

Amor Fati is a Latin phrase coined by the great philosopher Friedrich Nietzsche which translates to *"love of fate."* Nietzsche believed that we should accept our fate, both the good and the bad, without resentment and use it to move ahead in life.

This idea may seem counterintuitive to many of us, especially when it comes to anxiety, a condition that often leaves us feeling out of control and overwhelmed.

But what if we could learn to embrace our anxiety rather than fight against it?

This is the fundamental basis of Acceptance and Commitment Therapy. ACT is based on the idea that our attempts to control our thoughts and feelings often lead to more suffering.

ACT focuses on accepting and being present in the moment while committing to actions that align with our values. The goal of ACT is not to eliminate anxiety or any other negative emotion but to help us live a meaningful and profound life even in the face of adversity.

ACT is rooted in six core principles:**acceptance, cognitive defusion, being present, self-as-context, values, and committed action**.

We will explore each of these principles in more detail throughout this chapter.

But before we do that, I want to leave you with a thought.

What if, instead of constantly trying to control our thoughts and feelings, we learned to love them and use them to propel us forward? What if we accept our fate, both the good and the bad, and decide to live using the life lessons we learn from it?

This is the essence of ACT, and I hope it will become a helpful tool in your journey of self-discovery and acceptance.

The History of ACT

Acceptance and Commitment Therapy (ACT) emerged on the psychological scene in 1986. It was pioneered by the esteemed psychologist, professor, and author Dr. Stephen Hayes.

Hayes developed ACT based on a combination of theories, including Relational Frame Theory, 1st and 2nd wave behavior theories, Existentialism, and Humanistic approaches.

When ACT was being developed, Cognitive Behavioral Therapy (CBT) was the dominant treatment approach for many mental health conditions.

ACT represented a challenge to certain core assumptions of CBT, including the belief that thoughts and feelings are symptoms and can be controlled. Instead, Hayes proposed that complex thoughts and feelings are daily and that the techniques people use to prevent or avoid them can ultimately lead to more suffering. In contrast to the methods taught by CBT therapists to reduce unwanted symptoms, ACT encourages individuals to learn to accept difficult thoughts and feelings while focusing on taking meaningful action in line with their values.

Society views negative" emotions as problems to be solved rather than standard parts of the human experience. Dr. Stephen Hayes argues that acceptance, mindfulness, and values are crucial tools for a transformative shift.

Instead of running away from our problems, we must face them head-on and commit to actions that help us embrace any challenge.

ACT combines mindfulness skills with the practice of self-acceptance to develop psychological flexibility.

ACT is based on Relational Frame Theory, a school of research that suggests the rational skills we use to solve problems may not effectively overcome psychological pain.

When we shift our thinking about pain, we can learn ways to live healthier, fuller lives.

Multiple comprehensive treatment manuals have been developed for using ACT to treat various mental health conditions, and research supports its effectiveness in treating substance abuse, psychosis, anxiety, depression, chronic pain, and eating disorders.

How ACT Works

The practice of Acceptance and Commitment therapy revolves around six core processes.

Acceptance

Acknowledging and embracing the full range of thoughts and emotions rather than trying to avoid, deny, or alter them.

Cognitive defusion

Distancing yourself from and changing how you react to distressing thoughts and feelings can mitigate their harmful effects. Techniques for cognitive defusion include observing an idea without judgment, singing the thought, and labeling your automatic response.

Being present

Being mindful in the present moment and observing your thoughts and feelings without judging or trying to change them, experiencing events clearly and directly can help promote behavior change.

Self as context

Expanding the notion of self and identity, recognizing that people are more than their thoughts, feelings, and experiences.

Values

Choosing personal values in different domains and striving to live according to those principles instead of acting solely to avoid distress or adhere to other people's expectations.

Committed action

Take concrete steps to incorporate changes that align with your values and lead to positive change. This may involve goal setting, exposure to complex thoughts or experiences, and skill development.

ACT aims to help individuals develop psychological flexibility, which is the ability to adapt to changing situations, accept unpleasant emotions, and act according to personal values. It is believed that clients can eventually change their attitudes and emotional states by taking steps to change behavior while simultaneously learning to accept psychological experiences.

During ACT therapy sessions, individuals may be taught how to apply these concepts to their life. They may learn to practice acceptance and cognitive defusion or develop a different sense of self distinct from thoughts and feelings. Sessions may also include mindfulness exercises designed to foster nonjudgmental, healthy awareness of thoughts, feelings, sensations, and memories that one has otherwise avoided. Therapists may also help highlight moments when actions did not fit values while assisting individuals to understand which behaviors would work better.

ACT is a highly individualized form of therapy, and the techniques and exercises used will vary depending on the person and their specific concerns.

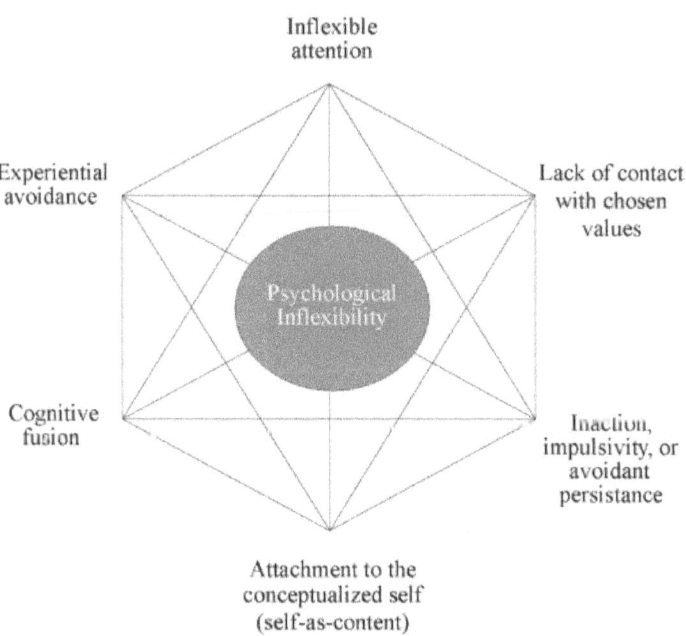

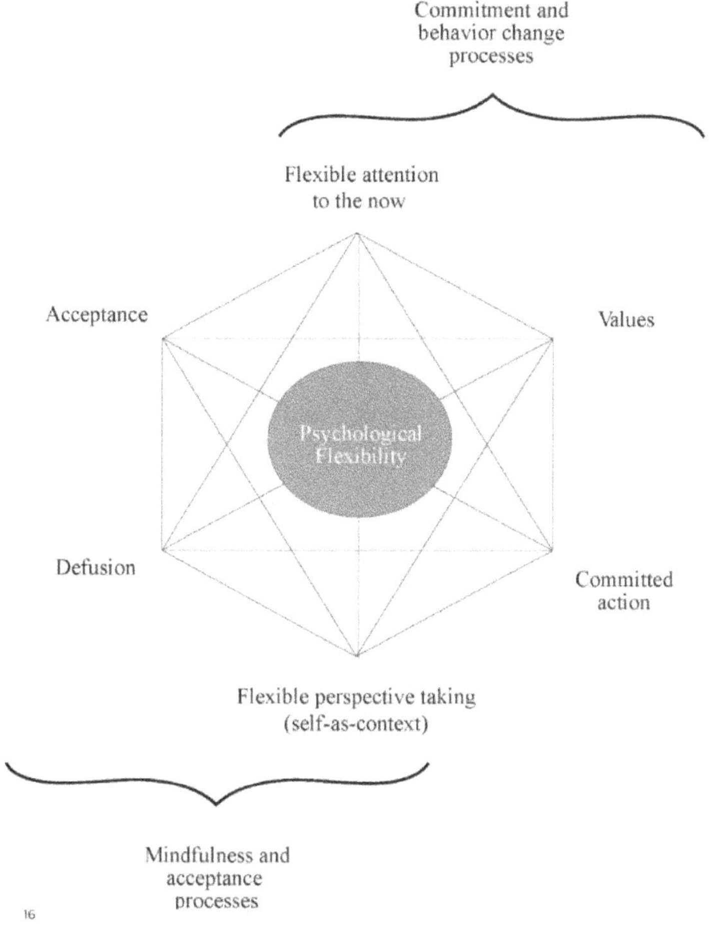

16

ACT and Mindfulness

Mindfulness and Acceptance and Commitment Therapy (ACT) are two critical components of the third wave of behavioral therapies that focus on developing mindfulness skills.

Mindfulness helps you to remain grounded in the present moment by paying attention to your feelings, physical sensations, and outside environment and offers you the benefits of peace, purpose, and happiness.

ACT differs from other mindfulness-based approaches such as Dialectical Behavior Therapy (DBT), Mindfulness-Based Cognitive Therapy (MBCT), and Mindfulness-Based Stress Reduction (MBSR) in many ways, such as being used with individuals, couples, and groups and having vast interventions to develop mindfulness skills.

ACT also does not aim for symptom reduction, as labeling an experience as a symptom can create a struggle. Instead, ACT aims to transform our relationship with complex thoughts and feelings so that we no longer perceive them as *symptoms* and perceive them as harmless, even if uncomfortable, transient psychological events.

It is important to note that ACT does not rest on the assumption of *"healthy normality,"* as a considerable percentage of the adult population suffers from a recognized psychiatric disorder.

ACT Reminders

For sufferers of anxiety, it's crucial not to become ensnared in a cycle of rumination. Individuals who struggle with anxiety and depression are particularly susceptible to getting trapped in this rabbit hole, which Acceptance and Commitment Therapy (ACT) aims to avoid through behavior modification. Rather than exacerbating negative thoughts, the first principle of ACT seeks to diffuse them.

An anxious brain is continuously vigilant, continually cycling through various scenarios in which things can go wrong or escalate. By allowing these emotions to pass through you, you can ultimately reach a place of calmness and tranquility on the other side of your thoughts, akin to a peaceful pond after a tumultuous storm.

It's important to remind yourself that even when you can't control your surroundings, you still have autonomy over your body.

Moreover, it's okay not to excel at everything you try. The point of testing is to learn and grow, and you can still derive joy from an activity even if you're not particularly good at it. Your strengths and weaknesses are valuable, as they offer unique opportunities for growth and development.

It's essential to resist acting on every single thought that crosses your mind. Allow them to flow by like a river, returning to their source.

Remember, whatever happened in the past is not happening right now. These are examples of the kind of self-talk an ACT therapist might encourage during these moments. Choose whichever ones resonate with you the most while you're practicing mindfulness.

Commitment is also fundamental to ACT and begins right from the first session. Changing your life is hard work, but acceptance and commitment therapy can gently guide you in the right direction.

Once you've achieved a sense of calm and clarity, you can take the necessary steps to achieve your goals.

Remember, commitment is a long-term endeavor requiring consistent effort and attendance. Show up for yourself, even when it's challenging, and keep pushing forward because you deserve to live a happy, healthy life.

ACT Exercises

ACT uses a range of experiential exercises and metaphors to help individuals understand and embrace their thoughts and feelings.

Stoddard and Afari (2014) expound in their book, *"The Big Book of ACT Metaphors,"* how they can be used to help teens with anxiety.

The Chinese Finger Trap

The Chinese Finger Trap metaphor is often used in ACT to help individuals understand the concept of psychological fusion. This is when we become fused or attached to our thoughts and feelings, and we believe they define us. The metaphor suggests that the harder we try to escape from our thoughts and feelings, the more trapped we become, just like how our fingers become trapped in a Chinese finger trap.

For teens with anxiety, this metaphor can help them understand that trying to avoid or suppress their anxious thoughts and feelings can make their anxiety worse. Instead, they can learn to accept their thoughts and feelings and let them be without becoming fused to them.

The Bus Driver

The Bus Driver metaphor is often used in ACT to help individuals understand the concept of values-based action. This is when we take actions that align with our values, even if they are difficult or uncomfortable. The metaphor suggests that our values are like a bus, and we are the bus driver. We can choose which direction to take the bus in, but we cannot control the weather or the traffic.

For teens with anxiety, this metaphor can help them understand that they can still take action toward their values, even if they feel anxious. It can also help them identify their values and take steps toward them, which can help them feel more fulfilled and less anxious.

The Weight of the World

The weight of the World metaphor is often used in ACT to help individuals understand the concept of experiential avoidance. This is when we try to avoid or escape from uncomfortable thoughts and feelings rather than accepting them. The metaphor suggests that carrying around our thoughts and feelings is like carrying a heavy weight. The more we try to avoid or escape from the weight, the heavier it becomes.

For teens with anxiety, this metaphor can help them understand that avoiding or suppressing their thoughts and feelings can make them feel worse in the long run. Instead, they can learn to accept their thoughts and feelings and let them be without trying to escape from them.

The Chessboard

The Chessboard metaphor is often used in ACT to help individuals understand the concept of cognitive defusion. This is when we learn to see our thoughts as simply thoughts rather than as facts or truths. The metaphor suggests that our thoughts are like chess pieces on a chessboard. We can observe and move them around, but we do not have to believe that they define us or our situation.

For teens with anxiety, this metaphor can help them learn to observe their anxious thoughts and feelings rather than becoming fused to them. It can also help them recognize that their thoughts are not necessarily accurate reflections of reality and that they have the power to choose how they respond to them.

Value Clarification Interventions

Value clarification exercises are designed to help clients identify and prioritize their values across various life domains.

Here are some example exercises you can easily do at home.

Personal Values Worksheet

This self-reflection exercise helps you examine different life aspects using ten categories. Write down what matters personally to you in the long run in each section. Think about why they matter to you and which you consider the most important. These can be values that you may consider unfulfilled. By completing this exercise, clients gain clarity on what they value most and can focus their attention and energy on those areas.

This worksheet has 10 categories:

- Romantic relationships – What sort of partner would you ideally like to be? How would you describe your ideal relationship? What kind of behaviors do you aspire to show toward a significant other?

- Leisure and fun – What kinds of activities appeal to you for fun? How would you enjoy spending your downtime? What's exciting for you? Relaxing?

- Job/career – What career goals matter to you? What kind of employment? Do you aspire to particular qualities as a worker? What sort of professional relationships do you want to develop?

- Friends – What social relationships do you consider important to develop? What do you think a critical social life to have? How would you like your friends to see you as a person?

- Parenthood – What kind of mother or father do you aspire to be? Are there particular qualities you'd like to role model for your kids? How would you describe your ideal relationships with them?

- Health and physical wellness – These questions will be based on fitness goals, aspirations, and the importance of personal health, physical well-being, and personal care.

- Social citizenship/Environmental responsibility – This category is about being part of the community and environmental aspirations and can include volunteer work.

- Family relationships – Like parenthood above, these values pertain to relatives like siblings, extended family, etc.

- Spirituality – Relevant questions here will concern religion and personal beliefs about anything meaningful at a more profound or more extensive level.

- Personal development and growth – Reflections in this category should relate to individual capabilities, competencies, skills, knowledge, and growth.

The 80th Birthday Party Speech

In this exercise, you imagine yourself as an 80-year-old looking back on your life. You can reflect on the type of person you want to be remembered as and write your 80th birthday party speech. The exercise encourages people to clarify their values and set meaningful goals that align with their desired legacy.

Experiential Avoidance - The Clean and Dirty Discomfort Diary

The difference between the ordinary discomfort that arises during living and encountering problems versus the discomfort that develops because of avoidance and control strategies is called clean versus dirty discomfort in ACT.

The Clean and Dirty Discomfort Diary exercise helps you recognize the experiential avoidance strategies undermining your goal achievement and behavioral change. The exercise will increase your self-awareness and mindfulness of the self-defeating consequences of avoidance.

The exercise distinguishes between clean discomfort, which includes unpleasant thoughts and emotions, and dirty discomfort, which provides for avoidant behaviors that are harmful in the long run.

You can appreciate this difference by keeping a clean versus dirty discomfort diary for a week.

This diary will help you pinpoint what triggers avoidance and your key avoidance strategies. Once you know these, you can use ACT interventions like defusion, mindfulness, and acceptance of discomfort to get you moving toward your values.

Over a week, use a table to record your responses each time you encounter complex thoughts or feelings.

Each time you experience such a situation in which you feel 'stuck' or where you are struggling with unwanted or challenging thoughts and feelings, complete one row as follows:

1. Describe the situation - what happened to cause your discomfort?

2. What was your initial reaction? What did you think or feel? What immediately 'showed up' in thoughts, feelings, and sensations?

3. On a scale of 1 to 10 where 0 = none and 10 = extreme, what was your level of distress?

4. What actions did you take to avoid the discomfort? Did you struggle with things you didn't like? Did you criticize or bully yourself? Did you try to shove your reactions back or pretend they weren't there? Did you try to distract yourself with food, alcohol, smoking, TV, etc.?

5. On a scale of 1 to 10, where 0 = none and 10 = extreme, how did your distress level change after your distractive action?

Circles of Influence

Values are the ideals most important to you in life. These may include things like love, respect, or empathy. Values play a role in shaping your goals, priorities, and even your identity. They are influenced by personal beliefs, as well as by your family, friends, and society. Acting per your values can help you achieve a happier life.

This exercise can help you explore how other people influence your values and what unique values they hold.

List 5 values in a circle that pertain to you, your family, your friends, and society. Self-reflect after completing this exercise by asking the following questions.

- How and when were your top values formed?

- What person or people most influenced your values?

- How are your values similar to and different from those of others?

- How do your values play a role in your everyday life?

The Benefits of ACT

ACT has shown great promise in helping individuals develop greater psychological flexibility, improving overall well-being.

What is Psychological Flexibility?

Psychological flexibility is adapting and responding effectively to different situations and circumstances, including those that may cause stress, anxiety, or depression. It involves embracing thoughts and feelings when they are helpful and letting them go when they are not, rather than being controlled by them.

The Benefits of ACT in Enhancing Psychological Flexibility

ACT is unique in its focus on psychological flexibility. By teaching clients to accept and embrace their thoughts and feelings rather than trying to suppress or avoid them, ACT helps clients develop greater psychological flexibility.

Let me explain how it works:

Reduces Anxiety and Depression Symptoms

ACT has been shown to reduce symptoms of anxiety and depression by enhancing psychological flexibility. Clients learn to accept their thoughts and feelings rather than trying to avoid or suppress them, which can reduce symptoms.

Improves Quality of Life

ACT also aims to help clients live a more meaningful life. Clients can experience a greater sense of purpose and fulfillment by clarifying their values and acting according to those values. This leads to an improved overall quality of life.

Enhances Coping Skills

ACT provides clients practical skills and strategies for coping with difficult emotions and experiences. Clients learn to respond to their thoughts and feelings more adaptively, which can help them navigate challenging situations with greater ease.

Builds Resilience

Clients can also develop greater resilience by developing greater psychological flexibility. This means they are better equipped to handle stress and adversity, returning from difficult experiences with greater ease.

The Pros and Cons of ACT

Despite the benefits that Acceptance and Commitment Therapy renders for each client, it is fairly important to consider the limitations of the therapy and recognize that it may not be the best fit for everyone.

Ultimately, individuals and their healthcare providers should work together to determine the best course of treatment for their unique needs.

Here are some pros and cons of ACT:

Pros of ACT

Broad Effcctivcncss

Research has shown that ACT is effective at treating a variety of mental health conditions, including anxiety, depression, OCD, chronic pain, and more.

Improved Quality of Life

ACT not only helps individuals deal with symptoms of mental health conditions but can also improve overall quality of life by promoting psychological flexibility.

Unique Approach

ACT is part of the "third wave" of psychotherapies, focusing on mindfulness, acceptance, and values-based living. This approach may resonate with individuals who have not benefited from other types of therapy.

Cons of ACT Therapy

Limited Research

While early studies on the effectiveness of ACT are promising, more research is needed to fully understand its efficacy, particularly in comparison to other forms of therapy.

Similarity to Other Therapies

Some critics argue that ACT is too similar to other forms of therapy, especially CBT, and may not represent a significantly different approach.

Not a One Size Fits All

While ACT can effectively treat mental health conditions, it may not be the right fit for every individual and may not be a cure-all solution.

ACT and Teenage Anxiety

Let's consider a teenage student Divya, who struggles with anxiety. She constantly worries about her schoolwork, social life, and future. She often beats herself up for her mistakes and dwells on her failures, making her feel stuck and unable to progress. Her parents are concerned about her well-being and want to find a solution to help her break free from this cycle of negative thinking.

For a teenager like Aliza, navigating the complexities of life can be overwhelming. Teens have too much pressure to fit in and succeed. It's easy to get trapped in a cycle of self-doubt and negativity. ACT provides a safe space for teens to explore their thoughts and feelings without fearing judgment or criticism.

So, how does ACT work for teens?

A vital component of ACT is learning to accept complex thoughts and feelings rather than avoiding them. This can be especially valuable for teenagers and adolescents prone to self-criticism or negative self-talk. When they learn to accept their thoughts and feelings without judgment, they can feel more in control and empowered to take positive action toward their goals.

ACT also emphasizes the importance of values-based action, or actions that align with one's values and goals. This can help teenagers and adolescents focus on what is truly important to them rather than getting bogged down in worries or fears about the future.

ACT can be beneficial for teens struggling to process their emotions. As teenagers navigate the challenges of growing up, they may encounter painful memories and fears about the future that can trigger anxiety. ACT provides language and experiential exercises that teach teens to accept and manage these difficult thoughts and emotions, helping them move forward and make positive changes in their lives.

ACT teaches teens to accept their thoughts and feelings rather than trying to suppress them. This acceptance helps to reduce the power that negative thoughts and emotions have over their lives. Through various exercises, such as values-oriented behavior and mindfulness practices, teens learn to observe their thoughts and feelings without judgment while developing greater self-awareness and self-compassion. They then know how to use this newfound awareness to commit to their values and goals rather than being held back by their anxiety.

ACT uniquely provides language and experiential exercises to help individuals learn how to access and accept their thoughts and feelings. These exercises can benefit teenagers who struggle with expressing themselves or understanding their emotions. When they know how to accept their experiences, teens can learn to avoid unhealthy coping mechanisms like drug and alcohol use.

Parents may also benefit from learning about ACT and how it can help their anxious teenagers. They better understand their child's struggles and the tools available to help them so parents can provide invaluable support and guidance. With its evidence-based approach and proven results, ACT is a compelling option for families seeking effective treatment for teenage anxiety.

Research has shown that ACT can be highly effective for teenagers and adolescents struggling with anxiety. A study published in the Journal of Contextual Behavioral Science found that ACT effectively improved emotional regulation in teenagers with emotional and behavioral difficulties (Harnett et al., 2015).

Another study published in the Trials Journal found that ACT was effective in reducing anxiety symptoms in a group of adolescents. The study used a randomized controlled design, meaning that some participants received ACT while others received traditional or no therapy. The results showed that the ACT group significantly reduced anxiety symptoms compared to the other groups.

A study published in the Journal of Contextual Behavioral Science found that ACT effectively reduced anxiety symptoms in a group of college students. The study used a pre-test/post-test design, meaning participants completed assessments before and after receiving ACT. The results showed that the ACT group had significant reductions in anxiety symptoms, as well as improvements in overall psychological flexibility.

Studies have shown that ACT can be particularly effective for teens with anxiety. For example, Swain et al., (2015) conducted a systematic review of intervention studies and found that ACT significantly improved anxiety symptoms among children and adolescents. Halliburton and Cooper (2015) similarly found that ACT could be adapted for use with teens and that it had the potential to be a valuable addition to standard treatment approaches.

ACT can also be beneficial for teens struggling with chronic pain. In a study of adolescents with chronic pain, those who participated in an ACT intervention reported significant improvements in their pain intensity, physical function, and emotional well-being. ACT effectively treats eating disorders in adolescents, with one study finding that it improved eating disorder symptoms and body image concerns.

If you or someone you know is struggling with anxiety, consider speaking to a therapist trained in ACT to see if this approach could be helpful for you.

How to Find an ACT Therapist

To find an Acceptance and Commitment Therapist, look for a licensed mental health professional with additional training in ACT.

Several mental health professionals may offer ACT, including psychiatrists, psychologists, social workers, or mental health counselors.

Ask about the therapist's training background and experience with ACT, and seek referrals from organizations such as the Association for Contextual Behavioral Science (ACBS) or the Association for Behavioral and Cognitive Therapies (ABCT).

Look for a therapist who is an active, empathic listener and an active guide. ACT sessions tend to be hands-on, often including psychological exercises or mindfulness training, as well as homework after the session is done. Completing these exercises is an integral part of ACT, as this is how you can learn new skills and improve your psychological flexibility.

The therapist should also discuss your values and goals during therapy. ACT works well in various therapy formats: face-to-face sessions, guided online courses, or even interactive apps.

Sessions typically last from 30 to 60 minutes and may occur over 6 to 12 weeks.

I hope by now you understand that Acceptance and Commitment Therapy (ACT) offers a unique and practical approach for teenagers and adolescents struggling with anxiety.

ACT focuses on acceptance, mindfulness, and committing to valued goals. It helps individuals develop psychological flexibility and healthier coping methods with challenging emotions and situations.

Finding the right ACT therapist may take effort, but it is worth the investment. Look for licensed mental health professionals with additional training in ACT, and don't be afraid to ask about their experience and credentials. The Association for Contextual Behavioral Science (ACBS) and the Association for Behavioral and Cognitive Therapies (ABCT) are excellent resources to help you find an experienced ACT practitioner.

So, if you are a teen struggling with anxiety or a concerned parent, take heart. ACT is a powerful treatment modality that can help you learn to live with more acceptance, mindfulness, and self-compassion.

With the guidance of a skilled ACT therapist and a commitment to practice, you can develop the skills you need to cope with life's curveballs and welcome growth and healing with open arms.

CHAPTER 9:

COGNITIVE BEHAVIORAL THERAPY

In this chapter, we dive into the fascinating realm of Cognitive Behavioral Therapy (CBT), a powerful tool that empowers you to reshape your thoughts, feelings, and actions.

As Albert Ellis beautifully stated,

"You have considerable power to construct self-helping thoughts, feelings, and actions and to construct self-defeating behaviors. You have the ability, if you use it, to choose healthy instead of unhealthy thinking, feeling, and acting."

Let us embark on this thought-provoking exploration of CBT, where we uncover the secrets to unlocking your inner strength and creating a positive and remarkable change in your life.

Imagine for a moment the immense power within you- the ability to shape your reality through the lenses of your mind.

Your thoughts, feelings, and actions are intricately connected, and with the proper guidance and understanding, you can transform them into allies on your path to well-being.

This is the essence of Cognitive Behavioral Therapy.

This is the power that lies within you.

CBT invites you to explore the dynamic interplay between your thoughts, emotions, and behaviors and empowers you to make conscious choices that align with your desired outcomes.

It is a collaborative journey where you, as the protagonist, work hand in hand with your therapist to uncover the hidden patterns and beliefs contributing to your anxiety.

Just as a skilled architect meticulously designs a blueprint for a building, CBT equips you with the tools to construct a new narrative; one built on healthy thinking, feeling, and acting.

It challenges the negative and self-defeating thoughts that often plague those struggling with anxiety, offering a fresh perspective that opens the door to growth and resilience.

Together, we will explore the core principles of CBT and discover practical techniques that can be applied in your everyday life. By examining the connections between your thoughts, emotions, and behaviors, we can identify unhelpful patterns and replace them with more adaptive alternatives.

The cornerstone of CBT is recognizing that our thoughts greatly influence our emotional well-being. The quote by Albert Ellis beautifully captures this notion, reminding us of our inherent power to choose healthy thinking over unhealthy patterns.

This chapter will delve deep into cognitive restructuring, challenging distorted thinking patterns, and cultivating self-compassion.

CBT goes beyond thoughts and feelings; it emphasizes the importance of action aligned with your values and goals.

We will explore various behavioral strategies to help you step out of your comfort zone, confront your fears, and build resilience. By engaging in gradual exposure exercises and setting achievable goals, you will learn to navigate the challenges of anxiety with newfound strength and determination.

It is important to note that CBT is an evidence-based approach, meaning that it is grounded in scientific research and is effective in numerous studies.

As we journey through this chapter, I will share with you the wealth of knowledge and research that supports the principles and techniques of CBT.

Rest assured that you are walking on a path that has helped countless individuals reclaim their lives from the grip of anxiety.

As we venture further into CBT, I encourage you to approach this chapter with an open mind and a willingness to challenge your existing beliefs.

Remember, you can shape your thoughts, feelings, and actions!

Together, we will uncover the transformative potential within you and set you on a path toward greater well-being and resilience.

Get ready to re-write your destiny!

A Brief History of CBT

In the 1960s, a brilliant psychiatrist named Aaron Beck made a remarkable observation while helping individuals with depression.

He noticed that these individuals exhibited specific patterns of thinking that weren't serving them well. Beck realized that our thoughts profoundly impact how we view ourselves, others, and the world around us. These thoughts influence our emotions and behavior, shaping our entire life experience.

Imagine it this way, if you perceive everything around you as pessimistic or threatening, it's no surprise that you'll feel pretty bad.

Our thoughts can color our perception and dictate our emotional responses. This is where the concept of cognitive distortions comes into play. These distortions are like "mind tricks" that warp our thinking, leading to negative emotions and unhelpful behaviors.

The fundamental principle underlying Cognitive Behavioral Therapy (CBT) is that most emotional and behavioral reactions are learned, which means they can be unlearned or changed.

Unlike other forms of therapy that delve deeply into past traumas or life history, CBT primarily focuses on the present and the thoughts and events shaping your current experience of anxiety.

Think of CBT as an umbrella term for a collection of therapies that share common elements.

Two of the earliest and most influential forms of CBT are *Rational Emotive Behavior Therapy* (REBT), developed by the remarkable Albert Ellis in the 1950s, and *Cognitive Therapy*, pioneered by Aaron T. Beck in the 1960s.

Both REBT and Cognitive Therapy rest on the belief that mental illnesses stem from faulty cognitions, faulty ways of thinking about ourselves, others, and the world. These faulty thoughts can manifest as cognitive deficiencies, such as a lack of planning, problem-solving skills, or cognitive distortions, where we process information inaccurately.

To put it simply, these faulty cognitions cause distortions in how we perceive things. Ellis believed that irrational thinking was the culprit, while Beck proposed the concept of the cognitive triad, which involves distorted views of ourselves, the world, and the future.

In CBT, therapists guide clients through evaluation, helping them identify and challenge their distorted cognitions. Clients learn to distinguish between their thoughts and reality, recognizing the powerful influence that thoughts have on their emotions and behavior. They're taught to observe and monitor their thoughts, gaining greater awareness of how these thoughts contribute to their anxiety.

But CBT isn't just about thoughts. It also incorporates behavioral interventions. Therapists assign homework assignments, like keeping a thought diary or engaging in specific tasks that challenge irrational beliefs. Through these exercises, clients uncover the unhelpful assumptions underpinning their anxiety, and, importantly, they get to prove these beliefs wrong.

Let's illustrate this with an example.

Imagine a teenager who experiences anxiety in social situations. They might believe that they're constantly being judged or that others see them as awkward or unlikeable. As part of their CBT treatment, their therapist might assign them homework: *meet a friend at a local restaurant for breakfast.*

Initially, the teenager might feel incredibly anxious about the prospect of socializing in a restaurant setting. But by challenging their irrational beliefs and engaging in the activity, they can gather evidence that contradicts their anxious thoughts.

Perhaps they discover that their friend genuinely enjoys their company and that others at the restaurant are accepting and friendly. Over time, these experiences and alternative perspectives gradually reshape their beliefs, reducing anxiety and increasing confidence.

Albert Ellis, the brilliant mind behind Rational Emotive Behavior Therapy (REBT), emphasized changing irrational beliefs to more rational ones.

He believed that each of us holds unique assumptions about ourselves and the world, guiding our actions and influencing how we respond to various situations.

According to Ellis, other common irrational assumptions can contribute to anxiety:

- The belief that one must excel in everything they do, leading to excessive self-criticism and fear of failure.

- The belief that it is catastrophic when things don't go exactly as desired, causing immense distress and an inability to cope with setbacks.

- The belief that happiness solely depends on external circumstances or other people's actions, leaving individuals feeling powerless and disempowered.

- The belief that one must rely on someone stronger or more capable than themselves, leading to dependence and a lack of self-confidence.

- The belief that past experiences and history have an overwhelming influence on the present life, limiting individuals from embracing new possibilities and growth.

- The belief that there is a perfect solution to every problem, and if it's not found, it's a complete disaster, creating immense pressure and anxiety.

Ellis recognized that individuals often cling forcefully to these illogical ways of thinking. He employed highly emotive techniques in REBT to help them break free from these irrational beliefs.

Individuals are encouraged to challenge and change their irrational thinking patterns through vigorous and forceful interventions.

The ABC model is a powerful tool used in cognitive therapy, including REBT.

This technique helps individuals understand the connection between activating events, their beliefs, and the following emotional and behavioral consequences.

In the ABC model:

A represents the Activating Event or the objective situation that triggers a strong emotional response or negative thinking.

B stands for Beliefs, where individuals identify and write down the negative thoughts that arise in response to the activating event.

C represents the Consequence, which includes the negative feelings and dysfunctional behaviors that result from the thoughts identified in column B.

Ellis argued that it's not the activating event that directly causes negative emotional and behavioral consequences. Instead, the interpretation of the event through irrational beliefs drives these consequences.

To provide an example, let's consider a teenager with social anxiety.

Suppose they receive an invitation to a party. The party (the activating event) triggers thoughts such as *"I'll embarrass myself," "Nobody will talk to me,"* or *"Everyone will judge me."*

These negative thoughts contribute to feelings of anxiety (the consequence).

The therapist helps the teenager challenge these irrational beliefs through REBT by engaging in reality testing.

They may explore evidence contradicting these beliefs, such as instances where they've had enjoyable social interactions, or others have shown interest in their opinions. By questioning the validity of their negative thoughts, the teenager can form more rational and balanced beliefs, alleviating their anxiety and allowing them to engage in social situations more confidently.

Cognitive Behavioral Therapy empowers teenagers with anxiety to recognize and transform their irrational beliefs through the ABC model and other REBT techniques, providing them with the tools to navigate life's challenges with greater resilience and emotional well-being.

The Core Principles of CBT

There is an intricate connection between your thoughts, emotions, and actions, a beautiful tapestry woven together to shape your experiences.

CBT recognizes this interconnectedness and teaches us that how we think and feel about something profoundly impacts our behaviors.

It is a powerful realization that these thought and behavior patterns can be altered, providing a beacon of hope amidst the storm of anxiety.

At the core of CBT lies the understanding that psychological problems are not solely a result of external circumstances but rather are influenced by faulty or unhelpful ways of thinking.

Our minds can remarkably shape our perception of the world, and sometimes this perception becomes clouded and distorted by negative thoughts and beliefs. Similarly, learned patterns of unhelpful behavior can contribute to our struggles.

Empowering Change and Growth

The essence of CBT lies in the belief that individuals suffering from psychological problems can learn better ways of coping and managing their symptoms, leading to significant relief and enhanced effectiveness in their lives.

It is a beacon of hope, reminding us that we have the power within ourselves to challenge and transform our narratives.

The Cycle of Thoughts and Behaviors

Let us look at the intricate relationship between our thoughts, emotions, and behaviors, an interplay that can either elevate us or hold us back.

It begins with recognizing that inaccurate or negative thoughts and perceptions contribute to emotional distress and mental health concerns. These thoughts, in turn, often lead to unhelpful or harmful behaviors, perpetuating a cycle that can be difficult to break free from.

CBT offers a ray of light amidst this darkness. By learning how to address and change these patterns, we can effectively deal with problems as they arise, paving the way for reduced distress and enhanced well-being.

The power lies in shifting our mindset, challenging negative thoughts, and adopting healthier perspectives.

Unmasking Cognitive Distortions

In the realm of CBT, we uncover the concept of cognitive distortions, patterns of thinking that reinforce negative thought patterns and emotions.

These distortions manifest in various forms, such as filtering out the positive, engaging in polarized or black-and-white thinking, overgeneralizing, catastrophizing, and jumping to conclusions. They act as roadblocks on our journey toward resilience and peace of mind.

CBT offers a structured and tailored approach to identifying and addressing these cognitive distortions. Through collaborative work with a skilled therapist, you will gain insight into the thinking patterns contributing to your distress, paving the way for managing overwhelming emotions and transforming unhelpful behaviors.

Cognitive distortions, those pesky patterns of thinking that hinder our progress, are tackled head-on in CBT.

Let's take a closer look at some of these distortions, unveiling their detrimental impact on our well-being:

Filtering

This distortion leads us to focus solely on the negative aspects of a situation, disregarding the positive elements surrounding us. It's as if we're wearing glasses that only allow us to see the darkness, closing our eyes to the light.

Polarized Thinking/ Black-and-White Thinking

This cognitive distortion traps us in an all-or-nothing mindset, leaving no room for complexity or nuance. We may judge ourselves as total failures for not achieving perfection in one area, and failing to recognize that we all have growth areas.

Overgeneralization

Falling prey to overgeneralization, we base broad conclusions on a single incident or point in time. This leads us to believe that one setback defines our entire future, preventing us from embracing the possibility of growth and change.

Jumping to Conclusions

This distortion involves making unwarranted assumptions without any evidence. We convince ourselves that someone dislikes us without concrete proof or that our fears will materialize before we even have a chance to test their validity.

Catastrophizing/ Magnifying or Minimizing

Catastrophizing involves blowing situations out of proportion, expecting the worst possible outcome. Conversely, minimizing occurs when we downplay the positive aspects of our experiences, dismissing our achievements and desirable qualities.

Personalization

In this distortion, we believe that our actions have an exaggerated impact on external events or the behavior of others. We shoulder undue responsibility for the negative happenings around us, failing to recognize the complex web of factors involved.

Control Fallacies

Control fallacies lead us to believe that everything that occurs is solely a result of external forces or our own doing. It is important to acknowledge that there are factors beyond our control and to discern the boundaries of our influence.

Fallacy of Fairness

Life, as we know, is not always fair. This distortion arises from an excessive expectation of fairness in every experience, causing resentment and disappointment when reality doesn't align with our idealized concept of justice.

Blaming

Blaming others for our feelings or actions is a common cognitive distortion. It is essential to recognize that while others may influence us, we ultimately bear responsibility for our emotional well-being and choices.

"Shoulds"

The cognitive distortion of "shoulds" revolves around rigid rules and expectations we impose on ourselves and others. When these expectations are not met, we experience anger, guilt, or disappointment, disregarding the inherent complexity and individuality of human experience.

Emotional Reasoning

This distortion convinces us that our emotions reflect objective truth. If we feel unattractive or uninteresting in a given moment, we erroneously assume that we are inherently ugly or dull, failing to recognize the temporary nature of our emotions.

Fallacy of Change

Expecting others to change to suit our desires or assuming that our happiness hinges on external factors only sets us up for disappointment. We are responsible for our own happiness and personal growth.

Global Labeling/ Mislabeling

This distortion involves sweeping judgments based on one or two instances or qualities. We may label ourselves as total failures based on a single setback, failing to acknowledge our multifaceted nature.

Always Being Right

This distortion compels us to prioritize being right over fairness, empathy, or personal growth. It hinders our ability to acknowledge.

Heaven's Reward Fallacy

This distortion revolves around believing that any sacrifice or self-denial will inevitably lead to immediate and guaranteed rewards.

It's as if we expect the universe to operate on a cosmic balance sheet, rewarding us in direct proportion to our good deeds. However, life doesn't always adhere to such rigid principles. The reality is that our actions and their consequences are influenced by many factors, some of which may be beyond our control.

Holding onto the expectation of immediate rewards can leave us bitter and disillusioned when our efforts aren't met with the expected outcomes.

CBT Techniques

CBT offers a myriad of techniques that cater to your unique needs. Some of the most popular methods within the realm of CBT are as follows:

SMART Goals: Empowering Yourself with Purposeful Intent

SMART goals serve as guideposts on your path to transformation. They are specific, measurable, achievable, realistic, and time-limited. Together with your therapist, you will craft goals that empower you to transcend your current limitations step by step, leading to a more fulfilling and meaningful life.

Guided Discovery and Questioning: Challenging Assumptions, Embracing New Perspectives

Within CBT, the power of guided discovery and questioning emerges as a catalyst for personal growth. Your therapist will skillfully question your assumptions about yourself and your circumstances, encouraging you to challenge these thoughts and explore alternative viewpoints. Through this process of self-exploration, you will shed light on the unhelpful beliefs that hinder your progress, paving the way for transformative change.

Journaling: Unleashing the Power of Written Reflection

Your therapist may encourage you to jot down negative beliefs that surface throughout the week while inviting you to replace them with positive and empowering affirmations. Through this written reflection, you unearth the depths of your thoughts and emotions, transcending the confines of the mind and unleashing the power of self-expression.

Self-Talk: Transforming Inner Dialogue with Compassion and Constructiveness

The words we speak to ourselves hold immeasurable power. Within CBT, your therapist will guide you in exploring your self-talk.

What narratives do you weave within your mind? Are they laced with negativity and criticism, or do they embrace compassion and constructiveness?

Together, you will challenge and replace negative self-talk with affirmations that nurture and empower, fostering a more supportive relationship with yourself.

Cognitive Restructuring: Unraveling the Threads of Distorted Thinking

Cognitive distortions can weave a web of negativity and self-defeat. Through cognitive restructuring, you board on a journey of unraveling these threads, one by one. Your therapist will guide you in identifying cognitive distortions such as black-and-white thinking, jumping to conclusions, or catastrophizing. You will challenge these distorted patterns of thought and pave the way for a more balanced and realistic perception of the world.

Thought Recording: Unveiling the Truth Through Evidence-Based Analysis

This technique involves recording your thoughts and emotions experienced during specific situations and examining evidence that supports or contradicts your negative beliefs. Through this process, you gain a clearer perspective on the reality of the problem, allowing for the development of more realistic and empowering thoughts.

Positive Activities: Nurturing Positivity and Self-Care

Engaging in rewarding and pleasurable daily activities can be a powerful antidote to negativity and stress. Whether treating yourself to fresh flowers, indulging in your favorite movie, or taking a peaceful stroll in nature, these moments of self-care and joy can fuel your resilience and improve your overall mood.

Exposure Therapy: Confronting Fears and Cultivating Resilience

By gradually exposing yourself to distressing situations or triggers, you begin a journey of desensitization. Supported by relaxation techniques and coping strategies, you learn to navigate these challenging situations with increasing ease and reduced anxiety, reclaiming your power over fear.

Homework: Your Personal Practice for Growth and Mastery

Just as academic assignments deepen your understanding and proficiency in a subject, therapy assignments catalyze growth and mastery within CBT. Embrace these tasks because they empower you to participate in your own transformation actively. They provide opportunities to practice and integrate the skills you learn in therapy into your daily life. From replacing self-critical thoughts with self-compassionate ones to keeping a journal of unhelpful thoughts, these assignments foster familiarity and mastery of the tools at your disposal.

Common Goals in CBT

Forming New Habits: Cultivating Healthy Patterns of Thoughts and Behaviors

CBT aims to support you in developing new habits that align with your well-being and personal growth. When you replace old, maladaptive patterns with healthy and constructive ones, you pave the way for positive change and resilience.

Developing Interpersonal Skills: Nurturing Healthy Relationships and Communication

CBT equips you with the tools to develop interpersonal skills, fostering healthy communication, empathy, and assertiveness. These skills enable you to cultivate meaningful relationships and navigate social situations with confidence and authenticity.

Learning to Express Feelings: Embracing Authentic Self-Expression

We often find it challenging to express our emotions openly and authentically. CBT provides a safe and supportive space for you to explore and embrace the expression of your feelings. This is how you foster emotional intelligence and cultivate a deeper understanding of yourself and others.

CBT Exercises for Teens

Personifying the Bully

Imagine your anxiety as a schoolyard bully, whispering doubt and fear into your ear.

But here's the secret weapon: give that bully a name! Whether it's the Wicked Witch, Mean Machine, or Clumsy Clown, personifying your anxiety allows you to separate it from your true self.

This simple act empowers you to challenge and talk back to your anxiety, asserting your control over it.

Unmasking the Impact

To overcome anxiety, you must first understand its grip on your life. Uncover the chains that anxiety wraps around your dreams and aspirations. Create a map of what you avoid or can't do due to fear, such as sleeping in bed, visiting friends, or enjoying family meals. By shining a light on anxiety's influence, we gain the knowledge needed to break free.

The Power of Exposure Therapy

In our quest for victory, exposure therapy has become our trusted ally. Like a skilled archer aiming for a bullseye, we carefully design a "hierarchy of fears."

Imagine a series of challenges, each more manageable than the last, building your strength and resilience. Rather than thinking in absolutes, we ask you to consider degrees of difficulty.

Can you touch a doorknob with one finger? Open the door? By gradually exposing yourself to triggers, anxiety's grip loosens, and your sense of mastery grows.

Embracing the Scale of Fear

Let's take control of anxiety by assigning its numbers!

On a scale of 1 to 10, how difficult is it to write "vomit" if you fear being sick? Perhaps that's a 3.

Now, saying "I will vomit today" might be a 5, while seeing a cartoon of someone vomiting could rate a 7.

By rating your fears, you'll see they're not all as extreme as they seem. We'll dismantle anxiety's fortress brick by brick, proving that you can conquer your worries.

The Heroic Journey

You'll start in the safety of your room, gradually venturing into the outside world. Wearing silly hats or walking a banana on a leash might seem unconventional, but these brave steps lead to tremendous progress.

Remember, mastery takes time. Parents, you play a crucial role too. Do encourage your child to tolerate anxious feelings rather than rushing to protect them.

Thought Record Worksheet (By Psychology Today)

The Thought Record worksheet provides a template for clients to monitor their thoughts and emotions, evaluate their thinking, and explore adaptive responding.

It is constructive for clients experiencing negative or dysfunctional thoughts and feelings.

The worksheet has 7 steps:

1. On the far-left column, there is space to write down the date and time a dysfunctional thought arose.

2. The second column is where the situation is listed. Instruct the client to describe - in detail - the event that led up to the dysfunctional thought.

3. The third column is for automatic thought. This is where dysfunctional intuitive thinking is recorded, along with a rating of belief in the thought on a scale from 0% to 100%.

4. The next column lists the emotion(s) elicited by this thought, with a rating of intensity on a scale from 0% to 100%.

5. The fifth column is where the client will identify which cognitive distortion(s) they are experiencing regarding this specific dysfunctional thought, such as all-or-nothing thinking, filtering, jumping to conclusions, etc.

6. The second to last column is for the user to write down alternative, more positive, and functional thoughts that can replace the negative ones.

7. Finally, the last column is for the user to write down the outcome of this exercise.

Were you able to confront the dysfunctional thought? Did you write down a convincing alternative thought? Did your belief in the thought and/or the intensity of your emotion(s) decrease?

Thought Record Worksheet Directions:

When you notice your mood drops, take a moment to observe what thoughts are passing through your mind, and then jot these down in the Automatic Thoughts column. Then, complete the rest of the row (i.e., date & time, situation, and so on).

Date & time	Situation	Automatic thought(s)	Emotion(s)	Alternative thought(s)	Outcome
	What were you doing?	What exactly were you thoughts at the time? And how much did you believe each thought (0-100%)?	How did you feel at the time? And how intense was the emotion (0-100%)?	What evidence is there that the automatic thought is true? Is there an alternative explanation?	How much do you believe in the original automatic thought now (0-100%)? How do you feel now (0-100%)? What can you do now?

Pleasant Activity Scheduling

Worksheet

	Activity (Pleasure/Mastery)	Time (AM/PM)	Post-Activity Emotion Rating (0-100% pleasure or sense of mastery)
Monday	*E.g. Call a friend to chat (P)*	5 PM	70%
Tuesday			
Wednesday			
Thursday			
Friday			
Saturday			
Sunday			

Pleasant Activity Scheduling Worksheet (By Psychology Today)

The Pleasant Activity Scheduling worksheet is designed to help clients schedule enjoyable activities that they can look forward to.

Clients are instructed to write down at least one activity per day that they will engage in over the next week. This can be as simple as watching a particular movie or calling a friend to chat.

Activities can be anything the client finds enjoyable or pleasant, so long as it's not unhealthy (i.e., eating a whole cake in one sitting or smoking). You can also try scheduling an activity for each day that gives you a sense of mastery or accomplishment. It's great to do something pleasant, but doing something small that can make you feel accomplished also has beneficial effects.

This worksheet helps clients begin to design their life to increase everyday positivity and pleasure. The first two columns (Activity and Time) are to be completed in session, and the last column (Post-Activity Emotion Rating) will be completed by the client throughout the week.

Graded Exposure Worksheet (By Psychology Today)

Graded Exposure is a CBT technique that is designed to help people confront and overcome their fears. When people are fearful of something, they tend to avoid it. While this avoidance may help reduce feelings of fear in the short term, over the long term, it can worsen the fear.

Graded exposure involves creating a safe environment where clients can become "exposed" to what they fear and avoid. Exposure to feared objects, activities, or situations in a secure environment helps reduce fear and decrease avoidance.

The Graded Exposure worksheet includes 4 steps:

1. Make a list of feared situations that you tend to avoid. For example, someone with social anxiety may avoid making a phone call or asking someone on a date.

2. Rate each item according to how distressed you would feel if you encountered that situation on a scale from 0 to 100% (0 = not at all distressed and 100 = extremely distressed). For a person suffering from severe social anxiety, asking someone on a date may be rated a 10 on the scale, while making a phone call instead might be placed closer to a 3 or 4.

3. Rank items from most-feared (i.e., highest distress rating) at the top of the staircase to least-feared (i.e., lowest distress rating) at the bottom.

4. The staircase can now be used to guide the process of graded exposure.

Clients can be guided to start exposing themselves to the least-feared items, building up as more confidence is gained. Fundamental principles of exposure should be discussed (e.g., stay in a situation without escaping, attempt multiple repeats of each direction to encourage extinction).

Graded Exposure Worksheet
Worksheet

Construct a staircase with situations you tend to avoid because of fear or anxiety, with most-feared items at the top and least-feared items at the bottom. Rate each item according to how distressed you would feel if you encountered that situation, on a scale from 0 to 10 (0 = not at all distressed and 10 = extremely distressed).

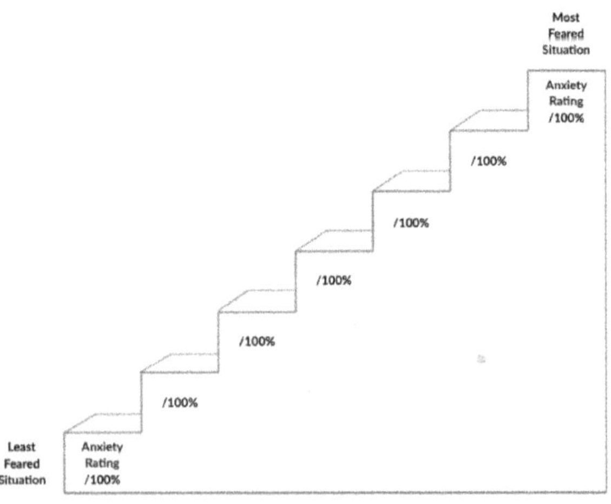

Advantages and Disadvantages of CBT

Cognitive Behavioral Therapy (CBT) is a widely recognized approach that offers numerous benefits for teens struggling with anxiety disorders.

It would help if you considered CBT's advantages and potential limitations to make an informed decision about whether it is the right fit for your teen.

Let's delve into these factors and explore what CBT has to offer.

Advantages of Cognitive Behavioral Therapy

1. Developing Healthier Thought Patterns

CBT provides a unique opportunity to gain awareness of negative and unrealistic thoughts that often contributing to anxiety. By actively engaging in therapy, individuals learn to challenge and replace these unhelpful thought patterns with more rational and constructive thinking. This shift in thinking can significantly impact emotional well-being and overall mood.

2. Effective Short-Term Treatment

One of the appealing aspects of CBT is its efficiency. Typically, positive changes can be observed within a relatively short period, ranging from five to 20 sessions.

Unlike other forms of therapy that may require long-term commitments, CBT offers tangible improvements within a manageable timeframe.

3. Versatility in Addressing Various Behaviors

CBT has proven effective in treating a wide range of maladaptive behaviors. Whether it's addressing anxiety, depression, or other psychological disorders, the principles and techniques employed in CBT can be tailored to suit different challenges.

This versatility allows therapists to adapt treatment strategies to match the unique needs of each individual.

4. Cost-Effective and Accessible

Compared to some alternative therapeutic approaches, CBT is often more affordable. Additionally, it can be conducted in various formats, including individual or group sessions, in-person or online.

This flexibility makes CBT accessible to a broader range of individuals, regardless of financial constraints or geographical limitations.

5. Development of Coping Skills

A significant advantage of CBT is its focus on equipping individuals with practical coping skills that extend beyond the therapy sessions.

Through active participation and practice, individuals gain tools to navigate and overcome anxiety-provoking situations in their everyday lives. This empowerment fosters long-term resilience and independence.

Disadvantages of Cognitive Behavioral Therapy

1. Commitment and Persistence

Engaging in CBT requires commitment and persistence. Success hinges on actively practicing the skills learned during therapy. Recognizing that progress may take time is crucial, and consistent effort is necessary for lasting results.

2. Suitability for Different Individuals

While CBT has proven effective for many, it may not be the best approach for everyone.

Individuals with brain diseases or injuries that impair their rational thinking may not benefit as much from CBT.

Also, if someone is not prepared to invest the effort and participate actively in treatment, they may not achieve the desired outcomes.

3. Potential Discomfort

Part of the CBT process involves addressing distorted thinking patterns and their associated emotions.

This introspective exploration can temporarily stir up or intensify emotional symptoms. Being prepared for potential discomfort can help individuals navigate this aspect of therapy more effectively.

4. Duration and Expectations

Although CBT is considered a short-term therapy, it's essential to understand that overcoming unhealthy thinking and behavior takes time.

Quick fixes should not be the primary expectation. Being patient and realistic about the duration of treatment can contribute to a more positive experience.

Evidence of Efficacy of CBT in Teen Anxiety

Several meticulously conducted studies have shed light on the undeniable benefits of CBT, reinforcing its position as a powerful tool for anxiety relief among teenagers.

Through personalized interventions, CBT empowers adolescents to conquer their anxiety, fostering resilience and paving the way for a brighter future.

Let's have a closer look.

Long-Term Relief

In their study, published in the Journal of Clinical Child & Adolescent Psychology, Seligman and Ollendick (2011) unveil a roadmap to anxiety relief. The authors diligently explore the effectiveness of CBT in treating anxiety disorders among young individuals. Through tailored CBT interventions, they discovered that anxiety symptoms significantly subsided. Notably, the benefits of CBT extended beyond the treatment period, providing long-term relief for adolescents battling anxiety.

CBT is a Gold Standard in Treating Anxiety in Teens

In a meta-analysis featured in the Journal of Clinical Psychiatry by Pegg et al. (2022), it is ingeniously synthesized that multiple randomized controlled trials confirm the true impact of CBT on anxiety symptoms in children and adolescents.

The findings affirm CBT as the gold standard in treating various anxiety disorders among teenagers. This formidable body of evidence underscores the reliability and consistency of CBT's positive outcomes.

CBT Improves Overall Functioning

A study by Kendall and Peterman (2015) provides an insightful overview of the evidence supporting CBT as a highly effective intervention for anxiety disorders.

It emphasizes the consistent findings that CBT reduces anxiety symptoms and enhances overall functioning in adolescents grappling with anxiety disorders. By targeting the underlying mechanisms of anxiety and equipping teenagers with coping strategies, CBT empowers them to navigate anxiety-provoking situations more effectively.

CBT targets teen anxiety by helping teens identify and challenge irrational thoughts, learn coping strategies, and gradually confront anxiety-inducing situations. By equipping teenagers with practical tools and techniques, CBT has demonstrated promising results in reducing anxiety symptoms and improving their overall quality of life.

To sum up, these studies collectively provide compelling evidence for the efficacy of CBT in teenage anxiety. CBT interventions tailored for youth have consistently yielded significant improvements in anxiety symptoms, with enduring benefits beyond treatment completion. CBT equips teenagers with the skills necessary to navigate anxiety-provoking situations successfully.

How to Find a CBT Therapist?

If you are considering CBT for your teenager or a teen battling anxiety, this guideline will help you navigate the process, from finding a therapist to understanding what to expect in a session.

Finding a CBT Therapist

To begin your CBT journey, follow these steps:

- Consult with your physician or explore directories provided by reputable associations to find licensed CBT therapists in your area.

- Consider your preferences, such as face-to-face or online therapy, to choose the format that suits you best.

- Check with your health insurance provider to see if they cover CBT and determine the number of sessions included per year.

- Make an appointment with your chosen therapist and mark it on your calendar to ensure you don't miss it.

What to Expect in a CBT Session

As you begin your first CBT session, here's a glimpse of what you can anticipate:

- Initial paperwork: You'll likely spend some time filling out forms related to privacy, insurance, medical history, current medications, and therapy agreements.

- Open discussion: Prepare to discuss the factors that led you to therapy, including symptoms and relevant personal history.

- Setting goals: Collaborate with your therapist to establish your therapy goals and communicate your expectations.

- Therapy policies: You'll review policies like confidentiality, session length, costs, and the recommended number of sessions.

- Questions and concerns: Don't hesitate to ask your therapist about combining medication with therapy, crisis management, their experience with similar concerns, therapy progress indicators, and what to expect in future sessions.

The CBT Experience

CBT sessions are typically structured, but your first appointment may have some variations:

- Assessment: Your therapist will inquire about your symptoms, emotions, and any physical manifestations of distress.

- Establishing rapport: Share any challenges, big or small, as therapy can help you address them effectively.

- Therapy logistics: Expect discussions on policies, costs, session duration, and the recommended number of sessions.

- Goal identification: With your therapist, define your therapy goals and what you hope to achieve.

- Open communication: Feel free to raise any questions or concerns during the session.

Remember that finding the right therapist is crucial. Stay committed, be open-minded, and actively participate in your sessions to maximize the benefits of CBT.

Whether you require a few sessions or a more extended treatment period, CBT offers an opportunity for profound personal growth and a path toward resilience and well-being.

Remember, the tug-of-war with anxiety is not easy, but it is worth every ounce of effort you put into it. As you navigate the world of CBT, know that you are not alone. There are therapists and professionals out there who are dedicated to helping you overcome the challenges that anxiety presents.

CBT empowers you to take charge of your thoughts, emotions, and behaviors. It provides the tools to reframe negative thinking patterns, confront fears, and build resilience. It's a journey of self-discovery and growth where you learn to transform anxiety into strength.

When you experience CBT, your progress is not measured by leaps and bounds but by small victories. It's about recognizing the moments when you challenge your anxious thoughts, face your fears, and emerge stronger on the other side.

Remember, it's not about eliminating anxiety entirely but about developing the skills to manage it and prevent it from controlling your life.

I urge you to keep an open mind and embrace the process. There may be setbacks and moments of frustration but know that they are stepping stones toward your ultimate triumph.

Surround yourself with a support system of loved ones who understand your journey and cheer you on every step of the way.

You are resilient, capable, and deserving of a life filled with joy and freedom.

Believe in yourself and trust in the power of CBT to guide you toward a brighter future.

Your anxiety does not define you; it is merely a part of your story that you can rewrite.

Your path to inner peace begins now.

Together, let us conquer our fears and unlock the boundless potential that lies within us.

You've got this!

CHAPTER 10:

THE ROLE OF A TEACHER

"*You wouldn't worry so much about what others think of you if you realized how seldom they do.*"

-Eleanor Roosevelt

These profound words behold a powerful truth that resonates deeply within the context of teenage anxiety.

As a teen, it's natural to find yourself preoccupied with the opinions and judgments of your peers. A teen often becomes entangled in a web of worry, fearing the spotlight of scrutiny and desperately seeking acceptance.

But let me share a secret with you-one that has the potential to liberate your mind and empower your spirit.

While it may seem as though the world around us is scrutinizing our every move, the reality is quite different.

The reality is that people are often too consumed with their own lives, worries, and insecurities to give much thought to their own perceived flaws and shortcomings.

The school environment significantly shapes a teenager's thoughts, emotions, and social interactions.

It is a place where a teen not only acquires knowledge but also navigates the complexities of social dynamics and self-identity. And while school can be a source of growth and inspiration, it can also become a breeding ground for anxiety and self-doubt.

Before we begin unraveling the intricacies of this chapter, I want you to know. You are not alone in this struggle.

The path to overcoming anxiety begins within the walls of your school, where compassionate educators stand ready to guide and uplift you.

Let us explore the landscape of the school environment and its role in teenage anxiety together and discover the invaluable support that awaits you within the embrace of a caring teacher.

School and Teenage Anxiety

Schools play a crucial role in the lives of teenagers, shaping their educational, social, and emotional development. However, it is no secret that school and stress often go hand in hand for many students, and anxiety at school has risen, especially since the onset of the Covid pandemic.

As more kids struggle with behavioral and mental health issues, high school anxiety has become a prevalent concern that needs careful attention and understanding.

Teenagers with anxiety disorders experience intense levels of anxiety that often manifest in physical and emotional symptoms. Unlike temporary anxiety over school, these feelings of tension and fear worsen over time and interfere with their daily activities. The impact extends beyond the individual, affecting their relationships with peers and family members. Parents need to recognize the signs of anxiety in their teens and seek expert assessment and support when needed.

Being a teenager has never been easy, and the modern world has only intensified their challenges. The rapid pace of technology, shifting social trends, and the demands of education can be overwhelming.

School, in particular, presents a challenging environment where teenagers navigate changes in friendships, romantic relationships, assignments, and extracurricular activities. While some anxiety is normal as teens anticipate the changes each school year brings, it becomes a concern when it becomes more pronounced and overwhelms or intimidates them.

There are various causes of school anxiety in teenagers, and it is vital to understand them to provide appropriate support.

Common Causes of School Anxiety

Academic Pressure

Increasing academic expectations, such as high-stakes exams, heavy workloads, and the pursuit of good grades, can pressure teenagers immensely. The fear of failure or not meeting expectations can lead to anxiety.

Social Concerns

Adolescence is a period of significant social development, and teenagers often experience anxiety related to fitting in, peer acceptance, and forming relationships. Bullying, social exclusion, or peer conflicts can contribute to school anxiety.

Performance Anxiety

The fear of public speaking, giving presentations, or participating in class discussions can cause anxiety in teenagers. The pressure to perform well academically or in extracurricular activities can exacerbate this anxiety.

Transition Periods

Moving from one school to another, transitioning from middle to high school, or starting a new academic year can trigger teen anxiety. The fear of the unknown, adjusting to new environments, and meeting new people can be overwhelming.

Test Anxiety

Exams and assessments can create significant stress and anxiety for teenagers. The fear of failure, the pressure to perform, and the anticipation of test results can contribute to school anxiety.

Bullying and Peer Pressure

Being a victim of bullying or experiencing peer pressure can harm a teenager's mental health and well-being. The fear of being targeted, humiliated, or ostracized by peers can lead to school-related anxiety.

Lack of Support

Insufficient support from teachers, parents, or classmates can contribute to school anxiety. When teenagers feel unsupported or misunderstood, their anxiety levels may increase.

High Expectations

Sometimes, teenagers may feel overwhelmed by the high expectations placed upon them by parents, teachers, or themselves. The pressure to excel in all aspects of school life, including academics, extracurricular activities, and personal achievements, can contribute to anxiety.

Time Management

Balancing multiple responsibilities, such as schoolwork, extracurricular activities, part-time jobs, and personal commitments, can lead to overwhelming anxiety. Poor time management skills and an overloaded schedule can contribute to school anxiety.

Negative School Environment

A school environment that lacks support, inclusivity, or safety can be a significant source of anxiety for teenagers. Factors such as harsh discipline, lack of resources, or a culture of competition can negatively impact a teenager's mental well-being.

It is crucial to be aware of the common symptoms to identify whether a teenager is experiencing school-related or separation anxiety.

Physical Symptoms

Stomachaches or digestive issues

- Headaches or migraines
- Fatigue or tiredness
- Difficulty sleeping or insomnia
- Rapid heartbeat or palpitations
- Shortness of breath or difficulty breathing
- Sweating or trembling
- Nausea or dizziness
- Muscle tension or aches

Emotional and Behavioral Symptoms

- Excessive worrying or fear related to school
- Irritability or moodiness
- Restlessness or feeling on edge
- Avoidance of school or specific school-related activities
- Difficulty concentrating or focusing on tasks
- Perfectionism or excessive self-criticism
- Excessive need for reassurance or seeking constant approval
- Tearfulness or frequent crying
- Social withdrawal or isolation
- Decreased interest or enjoyment in previously enjoyed activities

Cognitive Symptoms

- Racing thoughts or intrusive thoughts about school
- Difficulty making decisions or feeling indecisive
- Negative self-talk or self-doubt
- Catastrophic thinking or anticipating the worst outcomes
- Trouble retaining information or experiencing memory lapses
- Poor academic performance despite an effort
- Lack of confidence or low self-esteem related to school

Behavioral Changes

- Changes in eating patterns, such as loss of appetite or overeating
- Changes in sleep patterns, such as insomnia or excessive sleeping
- Avoidance of social situations or withdrawal from friends
- Increased reliance on unhealthy coping mechanisms, such as substance abuse
- Procrastination or difficulty starting and completing tasks
- Increased absenteeism or frequent visits to the school nurse
- Exhibiting signs of distress before or during school-related events.

Schools significantly influence young people's mental health, including those from diverse backgrounds and ethnicities.

For many teenagers, schools are not only educational institutions but also critical social environments where they form relationships and find a sense of belonging. Schools can positively impact mental health by promoting mental health literacy, providing access to mental health services, developing social-emotional skills, creating safe and inclusive environments, and fostering community and support for students and their families.

On the other hand, negative school experiences, such as bullying, disengagement from learning, dropout, and poor school transitions, have been linked to poorer mental health outcomes and social connections in young people.

Therefore, schools must prioritize strategies that enhance school connectedness. This includes nurturing positive relationships between teachers and students, creating a supportive and inclusive school culture, promoting student participation and engagement in school activities, and addressing the unique needs of students from diverse backgrounds and ethnicities.

It is important to note that school anxiety is not a recognized mental health diagnosis. However, it can be associated with several other diagnoses, such as depression, social anxiety disorder, generalized anxiety disorder, specific phobia, oppositional defiant disorder, and post-traumatic stress disorder. Therefore, a comprehensive and multidisciplinary approach is necessary to address school anxiety, involving parents or caregivers, teachers, mental health professionals, and school administrators.

Social Anxiety

Social anxiety disorder (SAD), also known as social phobia, is a common anxiety disorder that affects approximately one out of three adolescents between the ages of 13 and 18.

It is the most prevalent anxiety disorder and the third most common mental health disorder in the United States, with over 19 million individuals currently experiencing it.

Social anxiety disorder is characterized by an enduring and pervasive fear of social interaction, often leading to distress, self-consciousness, and fear of judgment in everyday social situations.

Individuals with social anxiety disorder may struggle to establish and maintain relationships and find their normal daily activities affected. They may also experience intense worry leading to social events, which can cause distress days or weeks in advance.

Understanding the Symptoms

Recognizing social anxiety disorder symptoms is crucial for teenagers and their parents. By identifying these signs, appropriate help and support can be sought.

Here are some common symptoms to be aware of:

Anxiety about being with unfamiliar people

Teenagers with a social anxiety disorder may experience heightened anxiety when interacting with individuals they do not know.

Difficulty engaging in conversations

Teens with a social anxiety disorder may find engaging in "normal" conversations with others challenging.

Self-consciousness and discomfort in social settings

Individuals with social anxiety disorder often feel self-conscious and uncomfortable in the presence of others, which can hinder their ability to socialize.

Embarrassment and fear of being judged

Fear of embarrassment is a hallmark symptom of social anxiety disorder. Teenagers may constantly worry about being judged by others.

Self-judgment and criticism after social interactions

Following social interactions, individuals with social anxiety disorder tend to engage in self-criticism, analyzing their behavior and fearing they may have misbehaved.

Fear and worry before public events.

Anticipatory anxiety is common among those with social anxiety disorder. Teenagers may experience intense fear and worry in the days or weeks leading to a social event.

Avoidance of social situations

Avoiding social situations is a common coping mechanism for individuals with social anxiety disorder. This avoidance can lead to diminished relationships and overall isolation.

Physical symptoms

Physical manifestations such as blushing, sweating, trembling, rapid heartbeat, stomach aches, nausea, and muscle tension may occur in social situations, even if they are considered *"normal"* by others.

Understanding the Risk Factors

While social anxiety disorder has no cause, several factors can contribute to its development.

Here are some common risk factors:

Genetic predisposition

Individuals with a family history of anxiety disorders may be more likely to develop social anxiety disorder.

Demeanor and temperament

Teenagers who are naturally shy, withdrawn, or apprehensive about new experiences may be at an increased risk of developing social anxiety disorder during adolescence.

Health or physical issues

Visible health or physical problems, such as physical deformities, visible scars, or birthmarks, can make individuals more susceptible to social anxiety.

Speech problems

Teenagers who struggle with speech problems, such as stuttering or speech impediments, may experience heightened self-consciousness and anxiety in social situations, leading to social anxiety disorder.

Traumatic experiences

Past traumatic experiences, such as bullying, humiliation, or social rejection, can significantly impact a teenager's self-esteem and confidence, potentially contributing to social anxiety.

Family or environmental factors

Growing up in an environment with high parental overprotection, excessive criticism, or rejection can increase the risk of developing a social anxiety disorder. Also, a lack of social support or limited opportunities for social interaction can contribute to social anxiety.

Negative social experiences

Repeated negative social experiences like being consistently excluded, mocked, or ridiculed by peers can develop a social anxiety disorder in teenagers.

Social Anxiety vs. Shyness

Shyness is a natural temperament, an inclination towards introspection, and a cautious approach to unfamiliar social encounters.

Shy teenagers may experience a sense of unease or discomfort when faced with new people or situations, often preferring to observe rather than actively participate.

While shyness may be seen as a gentle breeze, social anxiety disorder casts a more formidable shadow over the lives of some teenagers.

Unlike shyness, social anxiety disorder often disrupts daily functioning, hindering a teenager's ability to form relationships, pursue opportunities, and experience the fullness of life.

Teenagers from diverse backgrounds and ethnicities may face additional challenges when grappling with social anxiety disorder.

The intersection of cultural expectations, societal pressures, language barriers, and personal identity can amplify the fear of judgment, scrutiny, or rejection. Parents and caregivers must recognize and address these unique struggles with empathy and cultural sensitivity.

The Impact of Social Media on Social Anxiety

In today's digital age, social media has become an integral part of the lives of teenagers. It offers a platform for connection, self-expression, and information sharing. However, excessive use of social media can also contribute to developing or exacerbating social anxiety disorder in teens.

Comparison and Self-Esteem

Social media platforms often present an idealized version of people's lives, showcasing their best moments, achievements, and appearances. This constant exposure to carefully curated and filtered content can lead to social comparison and feelings of inadequacy. Teens may compare themselves to others, feeling they don't measure up in popularity, attractiveness, or success. This constant comparison can erode their self-esteem and intensify social anxiety.

Fear of Missing Out (FOMO)

Social media provides constant updates about social events, parties, and gatherings. Teens with social anxiety may experience a fear of missing out (FOMO) and feel immense pressure to participate in every social opportunity. This fear can trigger anxiety and increase their distress when they cannot attend or feel left out. The fear of missing out can further isolate teens and reinforce their social anxiety.

Cyberbullying

The online world can be a breeding ground for cyberbullying, with anonymity and distance providing a sense of safety for perpetrators. Teens who already struggle with social anxiety may become targets of online harassment, which can severely impact their self-esteem and exacerbate their anxiety in social situations. The constant fear of being judged or humiliated online can intensify social anxiety symptoms and lead to avoidance of online interactions altogether.

Limited Social Skills Development

Spending excessive time on social media can detract from face-to-face social interactions. Teens may become reliant on online communication and find engaging in real-life conversations and building meaningful relationships challenging. This lack of practice and exposure to in-person social situations can hinder their social skills development, making them more susceptible to social anxiety.

Strategies to Manage Social Anxiety in Teens

Encourage Open Communication

Create a safe and non-judgmental space for your teenager to express their feelings and concerns about social anxiety. Encourage young individuals to talk about their experiences, fears, and any challenges they face in social situations. Active listening and empathetic understanding can help them feel validated and supported.

Seek Professional Help

Consider consulting a mental health professional who specializes in anxiety disorders. A psychologist or therapist can provide effective treatments such as cognitive-behavioral therapy (CBT) or exposure therapy. These therapeutic approaches can help your teen identify and challenge negative thought patterns, develop coping strategies, and gradually confront their social fears.

Gradual Exposure and Skill-Building

Encourage your teenager to face their fears gradually, starting with low-stress social situations and progressively progressing to more challenging ones. Practice role-playing and offer guidance on effective communication and social skills. This gradual exposure can help them build confidence and develop strategies to manage their anxiety.

Limit Social Media Usage

Encourage your teenager to establish healthy boundaries with social media. Help them recognize its impact on their mental well-being and encourage them to take breaks from social media regularly. Encourage them to engage in activities that promote face-to-face social interactions, such as joining clubs, pursuing hobbies, or participating in community events.

Foster a Supportive Environment

Create a supportive network for your teenager by involving trusted family members, friends, or mentors who can provide encouragement and understanding. Building positive relationships and social support can help alleviate feelings of isolation and give a sense of belonging.

Encourage Self-Care

Emphasize the importance of self-care and stress management techniques. Encourage your teenager to engage in activities that promote relaxation, such as exercise, mindfulness, deep breathing exercises, or pursuing hobbies they enjoy. Taking care of their physical and mental well-being can help reduce anxiety levels.

Challenge Negative Thoughts

Help your teenager recognize and challenge negative thoughts and self-critical beliefs contributing to social anxiety. Teach them to identify irrational or distorted thinking patterns and replace them with more realistic and positive thoughts. This cognitive restructuring can help them develop a healthier mindset and reduce anxiety.

Teach Assertiveness Skills

Social anxiety can often be accompanied by difficulties in asserting one's needs and boundaries. Help your teenager learn assertiveness skills, such as expressing their opinions, saying no when necessary, and asking for what they need in social situations. Practicing these skills can enhance their self-confidence and reduce anxiety.

Encourage Social Involvement

Support your teenager in gradually increasing their social involvement. Encourage them to participate in activities or groups that align with their interests. This can provide opportunities to meet like-minded individuals and build social connections in a more comfortable and supportive environment.

Be a Positive Role Model

Model healthy social behaviors and coping strategies for your teenager. Show them how to confidently navigate social situations, handle rejection or criticism gracefully, and maintain a healthy balance between online and offline interactions. Your behavior can influence and inspire them to develop practical social skills.

Monitor Online Interactions

Keep an eye on your teenager's online activities and be aware of potential cyberbullying or negative influences. Teach them about online safety, responsible social media use, and how to handle any negative experiences they may encounter. Encourage them to block or report harmful individuals and seek support when needed.

Celebrate Progress

Acknowledge and celebrate your teenager's progress, no matter how small. Recognize their efforts to face their fears, take steps outside their comfort zone, and practice new skills. Positive reinforcement can boost their self-esteem and motivation to continue working on their social anxiety.

Remember that overcoming social anxiety is gradual, and setbacks may occur. Be patient and supportive throughout your teenager's journey. If their social anxiety significantly interferes with their daily functioning or causes severe distress, consider seeking professional help.

A mental health professional can provide tailored guidance and support based on your teenager's needs.

By implementing these strategies and providing a supportive environment, you can empower your teenager to manage social anxiety and thrive in social situations.

The Role of a Teacher in Teen Anxiety

Creating a culture of kindness and destigmatization within the school environment is crucial in helping students struggling with anxiety.

With the acceptance of mental health as an important aspect affecting the lives of children and adults, schools can adopt a proactive approach to addressing anxiety-related problems.

Let's explore the various ways teachers can counter teen anxiety and provide counseling for students.

Establishing a Culture of Kindness and Destigmatization

- Recognize the impact of mental health on students' lives and embrace a proactive approach.

- Encourage open discussions on social-emotional learning both at home and in school.

- Work collaboratively with parents to identify the source of anxiety, set goals, and implement strategies for managing anxiety.

Teaching Emotional Identification

- Conduct regular check-ins using a mood meter to help students verbalize various emotions.

- The red zone indicates the need for students to step away and calm down.

- Encourage students to express their feelings through writing and provide guidance to improve clarity.

Adjusting Classroom Policies and Practices

- Tailor classroom interactions to alleviate student stress.

- Accommodate students with anxiety about public speaking by allowing individual or small group presentations.

- Provide flexible seating arrangements to reduce the spotlight effect and help students focus.

- Offer verbal and written directions to prevent distractions and ensure equal participation.

- Give advance notice of upcoming presentations or tasks to allow students to prepare.

- Foster collaborative problem-solving and embrace mistakes as part of the learning process.

- Survey students at the beginning of the year to identify stress triggers and areas of concern.

Collaboration with Parents and Caregivers

- Maintain regular communication with parents to understand students' needs and progress.

- Prioritize parental involvement in addressing anxiety-related issues.

- Seek parental input in developing strategies for managing anxiety at home and school.

- Inform parents if a student is frequently absent, ensuring a smooth return to school.

Creating Opportunities for Temporary Escapes

- Promote mindfulness to help students regulate anxiety and redirect focus.

- Incorporate short yoga breaks or daily walks between classes to encourage relaxation.

Encouragement and Resilience Modeling

- Provide positive reinforcement that focuses on effort rather than outcomes.

- Highlight students' ability to embrace challenges and learn from mistakes.

- Model resilience by acknowledging and recovering from personal errors, helping students reframe their approach to obstacles.

Providing a Calm Environment for Maximum Potential

- Reassure students that mistakes and setbacks are standard in the learning process.

- Build confidence by praising their effort and recalling past successes.

- Be proactive in discussing complicated topics, such as divorce or global events, using age-appropriate language.

- Create structured routines, remove distractions, and allow time for breaks and rest.

- Remember, seeking professional help when needed is essential, and providing a calm environment can foster improvement in student well-being and academic success.

- Now, we'll discuss the various tools and strategies teachers can utilize to support students dealing with anxiety.

Breathing Exercises for Calming the Nervous System

- Incorporate simple breathing exercises into daily routines to trigger the body's relaxation response.

- Encourage students to take three slow, deep breaths during stressful moments to quiet the *"fight or flight"* response.

- Teach students the importance of mindful breathing and how it can be done discreetly without drawing attention.

Journaling for Emotional Processing

- Promote the use of journaling as an evidence-based tool for stress relief.

- Encourage students to write about their experiences, helping them interpret and make sense of their emotions.

- Emphasize the therapeutic benefits of regularly expressing emotions through writing.

Self-Care Strategies for Inner Calm

- Highlight the importance of sleep and good nutrition in alleviating teen anxiety.

- Encourage parents to support their teens in practicing self-care.

- Educate students about the connection between self-care and emotional well-being.

Positive Visualization for Stress Reduction

- Introduce the concept of positive visualization and mental imagery to enhance mental health.

- Guide students in visualizing positive outcomes and regulating their emotions.

- Show them how positive visualization can be a powerful tool for relieving stress and anxiety.

Yoga, Meditation, and Nature Connection

- Discuss the research-backed benefits of yoga and meditation in reducing stress and anxiety.

- Encourage students to explore these practices as tools for self-regulation.

- Emphasize the value of spending time in nature, as research shows it reduces levels of stress, depression, and anxiety.

Cultivating Strong Connections with Friends and Family

- Highlight the role of close friends in helping teens deal with anxiety.

- Encourage the development of authentic connections and guide forming of trusting friendships.

- Emphasize the importance of family time and open communication to support emotional well-being.

Personalized Stress Busters and Transition Support

- Engage in conversations with students to understand their specific needs and concerns.

- Encourage parents to ask their child or teen for input on what would support them in transitioning back to school more easily.

- Explore personalized strategies such as new outfits, after-school plans, or activities that boost confidence and reduce anxiety.

When To Seek Professional Help?

- Emphasize the importance of seeking professional help when anxiety symptoms persist or significantly interfere with daily life.

- Educate parents and students about the benefits of cognitive-behavioral therapy (CBT), dialectical behavioral therapy (DBT), and exposure-response therapy (ERP).

- Highlight the value of a collaborative team approach involving the child, parents, school personnel, and mental health professionals for effective treatment and management.

- Emphasize that mental health professionals can provide targeted support and coping skills for teens with anxiety.

- Stress the importance of early intervention to prevent the escalation of anxiety-related issues.

- Inform parents and students about the potential consequences of untreated anxiety, such as depression, substance use disorders, and social isolation.

As I conclude this chapter on managing teen anxiety, I want to assure you that help is within reach and that there is hope for brighter days ahead.

Anxiety can be a relentless bully, but armed with the right tools, strategies, and professional support, we can empower ourselves and our loved ones to overcome its grip.

Remember, teachers are not just educators but also compassionate allies who genuinely care about your well-being. They are equipped with various coping skills that can provide solace during distress. They can help you tap into your inner resilience and regain a sense of calm.

I cannot stress this enough, building a support network of trusted friends and nurturing connections with family members can be a powerful antidote to anxiety.

Surround yourself with individuals who understand and accept you; together, you can navigate the challenges of anxiety with greater strength and courage.

While these strategies can be invaluable, it is important to acknowledge that there are instances where seeking professional help becomes essential.

Mental health professionals possess the expertise to excavate more profound into the root causes of anxiety and provide tailored interventions such as cognitive-behavioral therapy (CBT) and exposure-response therapy (ERP). They are skilled in guiding you through healing and helping you regain control over your life.

I want you to know that you are not alone in this battle. Together, we will dismantle the barriers anxiety erects and create a future filled with boundless possibilities.

Remember, anxiety does not define you. You possess immeasurable strength within you, waiting to be unleashed.

You just need to let your light shine through!

The world eagerly awaits the remarkable person you are destined to become.

Stay resilient, stay hopeful, and know that you can conquer anxiety. I believe in you!

CHAPTER 11:

WHAT CAN PARENTS DO?

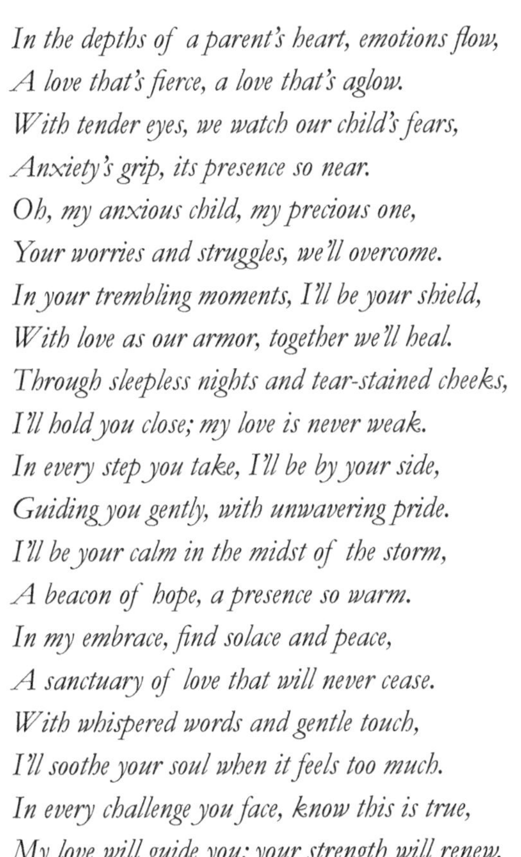

In the depths of a parent's heart, emotions flow,
A love that's fierce, a love that's aglow.
With tender eyes, we watch our child's fears,
Anxiety's grip, its presence so near.
Oh, my anxious child, my precious one,
Your worries and struggles, we'll overcome.
In your trembling moments, I'll be your shield,
With love as our armor, together we'll heal.
Through sleepless nights and tear-stained cheeks,
I'll hold you close; my love is never weak.
In every step you take, I'll be by your side,
Guiding you gently, with unwavering pride.
I'll be your calm in the midst of the storm,
A beacon of hope, a presence so warm.
In my embrace, find solace and peace,
A sanctuary of love that will never cease.
With whispered words and gentle touch,
I'll soothe your soul when it feels too much.
In every challenge you face, know this is true,
My love will guide you; your strength will renew.

You're not alone, my brave little star,
Together we'll conquer, no matter how far.
Through the highs and lows, my heart will stay,
A constant embrace, lighting your way.

Do you remember the day your child was born?

Do you remember how your heart was full of so much love that you thought it would burst out of your chest?

Do you remember how, then and there, you promised yourself that you would protect your child in every possible way?

As parents, we hold a profound responsibility for the well-being of our children. We strive to create a safe and nurturing environment where they can thrive.

However, when our teens experience anxiety or depression, it's natural to question our role and wonder if we have somehow failed them.

Feelings of guilt, embarrassment, and helplessness may overwhelm us. But let me assure you, dear parent, that you are not alone in this struggle.

Many factors contribute to teen anxiety and depression outside your control. For example, cultural pressures, the rapid advancement of technology, social instability, and even the confusion surrounding gender identity, to name a few.

Despite our best efforts, we cannot shield our children entirely from these influences. Similarly, we cannot control events that lead to depression, such as bullying, abuse, grief, and illness. As a parent, it's imperative to recognize that you are not to blame for these external factors that can significantly impact your teen's mental health.

However, it is also essential to acknowledge the role we may have played, even partially, in our child's struggles. Reflecting on our actions and words is a courageous step toward growth and healing.

If, upon introspection, you realize that you could have done things differently or provided more support, I encourage you to take the following approach.

Firstly, confess your shortcomings to yourself. Remember that no parent is perfect, and we all make mistakes. By humbling ourselves, we can find peace and the grace to move forward with solutions that help our children.

Secondly, consider confessing your mistakes to your child. Engage in an open and honest conversation, expressing your regret for any shortcomings and acknowledging your contribution to their struggles. This act of vulnerability can bring you closer together, demonstrating your humanity and fostering a deeper connection. It allows your children to connect with you on a level they didn't think was possible. It also provides an opportunity for growth and healing within your relationship.

Remember that mistakes, whether on your part or not, do not define the entirety of your parent-child bond.

Instead, focus on finding ways to seek help together. Encourage your teen to seek professional assistance from doctors and counselors.

Working collaboratively, you can explore practical means to support their journey towards improved mental well-being. This process of repair and reconciliation can transform what initially felt like a source of guilt and shame into a catalyst for personal and relational growth.

Research consistently demonstrates that parental involvement in their child's mental health treatment is directly linked to positive outcomes.

You have a unique position of influence as you interact with your teen daily. You can model and cultivate coping skills, providing them with invaluable tools to navigate the challenges they face.

The Critical Role of Parents in Teen Anxiety

Researchers specializing in childhood trauma and adolescent development recognize parents and caregivers as a vital link in addressing the urgent mental health crisis among teens.

The teenage years can be challenging for parents and adolescents, often marked by mood swings, risk-taking behaviors, and seemingly endless arguments. However, understanding parents' critical role in supporting their teens' mental well-being can pave the way for effective intervention and building healthier relationships.

Navigating the Storm: Understanding the Teenage Experience

During adolescence, teens undergo significant physical, emotional, and cognitive changes that can contribute to their vulnerability to anxiety.

Hormonal shifts associated with puberty and inadequate sleep due to early school start times can make teens irritable and more susceptible to stressors.

It's important to acknowledge that half of all mental illnesses emerge by age 14 and 75% by age 24, highlighting adolescence as a sensitive period for addressing mental health issues.

Parental Influence: A Powerful Risk Factor

Parent psychopathology emerges as a critical risk factor for anxiety and depression in youth.

Research suggests that children of anxious parents face two to seven times the risk of developing an anxiety disorder compared to children of non-anxious parents. Similarly, children of depressed parents exhibit rates of depression up to six times higher than children of non-depressed parents, often experiencing earlier symptoms. Various factors contribute to the transmission of psychopathology from parents to youth, including genetics, relationship dynamics, marital conflict, and modeling of maladaptive behaviors. Parents who struggle with anxiety or depression may unintentionally pass on these challenges to their children, impacting their mental well-being. (Yaffe, 2021)

Attachment Dynamics: Shaping Parent-Teen Relationships

Attachment theory provides valuable insights into the dynamics between parents and teens.

It suggests that emotional connection within a romantic relationship is a form of attachment, termed adult attachment. This theory extends to the parent-adolescent relationship, impacting the quality of attachment formed during this critical period.

Mothers with an avoidant adult attachment may exhibit indifference and rejection in parenting, lacking sensitivity to their adolescents' needs during stressful situations. On the other hand, mothers with an anxious adult attachment may display controlling and emotionally unstable interactions, struggling to provide stable support.

In contrast, mothers with secure adult attachment offer emotional stability and warm support to their children, creating a secure base from which adolescents can confidently explore their environment. A safe and supportive bond with a parent can serve as a haven for teens, reducing anxiety in stressful situations.

Family Dynamics: Systems of Influence

Family system theory suggests that a family comprises distinct hierarchical "energy" subsystems, such as the marriage and parent-child subsystems.

Energy generated within one subsystem can directly influence another, emphasizing the interdependence of family dynamics. For instance, the characteristics and functions of the interactions between spouses in the marriage subsystem impact the mother-child subsystem, affecting maternal psychological flexibility.

Maternal psychological flexibility refers to a parent's ability to accept negative thoughts, emotions, and impulses toward their adolescents while maintaining effective parenting behaviors.

Mothers with higher adult attachment avoidance and anxiety tend to employ rigid and strict parenting strategies. Consequently, adolescents undergoing rapid physical and mental development may not receive the flexible and practical support they need during stressful situations, exacerbating their anxiety.

The Mother-Adolescent Attachment: Nurturing a Secure Base

The mother-adolescent attachment represents the enduring and profound emotional bond established between mothers and their teenagers.

Maternal-adult attachment within the marriage subsystem significantly influences the quality of mother-adolescent attachment in the parent-child subsystem.

Mothers with avoidant adult attachments often exhibit evasive and indifferent responses, creating an unsafe relationship with their adolescents.

Conversely, mothers with anxious adult attachment tend to adopt controlling and unstable response styles, leading to an insecure attachment.

Comparatively, secure mother-adolescent attachment provides adolescents a safe space, offering psychological support during stressful situations and reducing anxiety. (Chen et al., 2021)

Parenting Styles: Impacting Anxiety Levels

Various parenting styles and practices can influence children's anxiety levels. Children and adolescents with anxiety disorders are more likely to be raised by non-authoritative parents, characterized by overprotectiveness, authoritarianism, or neglectful styles. These parents often exert exaggerated control, hinder autonomy, or employ harsh and inconsistent disciplinary measures. Such parenting approaches can contribute to heightened anxiety levels in children. (Yaffe, 2021)

Breaking the Cycle: Addressing Anxiety from a Family Perspective

Research demonstrates that anxiety tends to run intergenerationally within families, indicating a higher prevalence of anxiety disorders in families with anxious members.

Parents with anxiety disorders are seven times more likely to have children with anxiety disorders, resulting in increased anxiety-related problems for the entire family. Moreover, corporal punishment, including physical punitive measures, has been associated with elevated anxiety sensitivity and decreased sense of control among children. (Yaffe, 2021)

Matthewson et al., 2012 suggested that mothers' support, particularly in terms of companionship and informational support, may unintentionally contribute to daughters' anxiety levels. The study revealed an adequate relationship between mothers and lower levels of paternal anxiety was associated with lower state anxiety in sons. These findings emphasize the significant roles that both mothers and fathers play in protecting their children against stress.

Moreover, they suggested that the parent-child relationship with the opposite-sex parent may play a crucial role in alleviating anxiety in children.

Bögels and Phares (2008) proposed a compelling theory on the distinct roles mothers and fathers may play in protecting their children against anxiety at different stages of child development.

They suggested that fathers can protect infants through play and encouraging appropriate risk-taking behaviors, while mothers offer warm care and protection.

Fathers can facilitate their child's social integration and independence in the pre-adolescent stage, while mothers foster close personal relationships and social network development. In adolescence, fathers promoting independence and mothers allowing their adolescents to transition to the outside world act as safeguards against anxiety-related problems.

Parental Contribution To Teen Anxiety

So, what might be the ways parents are exacerbating their child's anxiety?

Let's have a look.

Overprotection: The Caged Bird Syndrome

Consider a parent who wraps their child in an impenetrable cocoon, shielding them from every conceivable hardship.

On the surface, it may seem like an act of love and protection, but beneath lies the breeding ground for anxiety to flourish. Parents inadvertently hinder teens' development of resilience and coping mechanisms by sheltering them from life's inevitable challenges and discomfort.

Remember, my dear parents, the caged bird may feel safe, but it denies the opportunity to soar and conquer the vast skies of life.

Constant Reassurance: Fueling the Anxiety Flame

"Oh, my dear child, everything will be fine. Don't worry."

While these words emanate from a place of love and concern, they can inadvertently fan the flames of anxiety. Constant reassurance, though well-intentioned, may unintentionally reinforce the belief that the world is treacherous, perpetuating an anxiety-driven cycle of seeking external validation.

Instead, consider fostering a sense of self-reliance and inner strength within your teen. Encourage them to face their fears and uncertainties with courage, knowing they are resilient enough to weather life's storms.

High Expectations: The Perfectionist's Plague

As parents, we yearn for our children to excel, surpass our accomplishments, and shine brightly in the realm of success. In short, we want them to be perfect.

However, beware of the perils of unrelenting expectations. When the bar is set impossibly high, it gives anxiety a chance to thrive. The fear of failure and the constant pursuit of perfection can erode self-esteem and ignite a never-ending cycle of anxiety-driven self-criticism.

Embrace the beauty of imperfection and nurture a supportive environment where mistakes are seen as valuable stepping stones toward growth and self-discovery.

Emotional Contagion: The Ripple Effect

Parents, you need to recognize the immense power of your emotions and their profound impact on your beloved teens.

When you navigate the world wearing the heavy cloak of anxiety, your child absorbs it like a sponge. Emotional contagion is real and can perpetuate a cycle of heightened anxiety within the family unit.

Seek comfort in your well-being and invest in self-care and emotional resilience. By cultivating your inner peace, you create a nurturing environment for your teen to reflect upon and learn the art of emotional regulation.

Communication Breakdown: The Unheard Cry

In the hustle and bustle of our modern lives, it is easy to overlook the power of authentic and empathetic dialogue. Often, parents unwittingly dismiss or invalidate their teen's anxieties, brushing them off as trivial or unwarranted. Remember, my dear parents, your teen's anxiety is their reality and demands compassionate understanding.

Open your hearts and create a safe space for open conversations. Embrace active listening, be free from judgment, and offer unwavering support.

Together, you can win the tug of war with anxiety.

Towards a Path of Healing and Support

Recognizing the critical role of parents in teen anxiety is the first step toward promoting emotional well-being in adolescents.

By understanding the influence of parental factors, attachment dynamics, family systems, and parenting styles, parents can effectively develop strategies to support their teens.

Open communication, empathetic listening, and a secure and nurturing environment can nurture a healthier parent-teen relationship, promoting resilience and emotional growth in adolescents. Seeking professional guidance and counseling can also offer valuable tools and techniques for parents and teens to navigate the challenges of anxiety together.

Here are some practical tips and tricks you can use to support your anxious teen:

Tip 1: Respond to their anxiety in the right way

When your teenager expresses anxiety, it's crucial to respond in a calm and hopeful manner. Start by having open conversations with your child, inviting them to express their feelings and worries. Instead of dismissing their concerns, reassure them that it's normal to feel scared and let them know you are here to support them every step of the way.

To help your child articulate their feelings, encourage them to communicate through storytelling. By stepping outside themselves, they may feel more comfortable describing their emotions. This storytelling approach can create a safe space for them to open up.

Your response should express concern and understanding, showing empathy and compassion.

Research suggests that maternal empathy significantly alleviates distress in children. Let your child know that anxiety is nothing to be ashamed of and that you're there to help them understand their anxiety triggers and find ways to manage them. By adopting a teamwork approach, you build a bond with your child and nurture their ability to tolerate anxiety.

While being supportive, it's essential not to be overly controlling. Avoid overprotectiveness, as it can hinder your child's ability to manage anxiety.

Instead, provide attentive listening and empathy, which already offer valuable support. Engage in conversations about different situations and help your child develop strategies to handle them.

For example, if your child experiences separation anxiety at a friend's house, brainstorm appropriate responses together, such as asking about pick-up times or requesting a call to confirm arrival. These strategies can reassure your child and reduce anxiety.

Focus on building your child's coping skills. Instead of avoiding anxiety triggers, assist them in developing effective coping strategies. Frequent positive feedback will encourage their self-confidence.

Set small, achievable goals and acknowledge their efforts and progress as you proceed. If setbacks occur, reassure your child of their learning experiences, empowering them to take control of future situations.

Tip 2: Be a positive role model for your child

Your behavior and attitude greatly influence your teenager's ability to manage stress and anxiety. Your child looks up to you for guidance, so it's important to model healthy coping strategies. Aim to remain calm and patient when dealing with problems or challenging situations. How you speak and what you speak about can profoundly impact your teenager's values and behavior. Be what you want your child to learn.

Taking care of yourself is also crucial. Prioritize sufficient sleep, regular exercise, and a healthy diet, as these practices can inspire your child to do the same. Engage in activities like yoga, meditation, or other relaxation techniques, showing your children the importance of well-being.

Be mindful of negative comments about your body, which can contribute to poor self-image and body shaming.

You teach your children valuable lessons by modeling a healthy approach to life. Emphasize that everyone makes mistakes, including parents, and highlight the importance of resilience in overcoming adversity. When your children witness you going through the same struggles and handling them with effective and practical strategies, it alleviates unnecessary pressures.

Tip 3: Practice relaxation techniques with your child

Offer to engage in relaxation exercises with your teenager, acknowledging their feelings and providing proactive strategies.

Deep breathing and meditation exercises can be powerful tools for anxiety relief. Teach your child deep belly breathing, where they place one hand on their chest and the other on their belly. Inhaling should expand the belly, and exhaling should contract it.

Encourage mindful breathing, where your child focuses on their breath and brings attention to the present moment. This can help shift their focus away from anxious thoughts and promote a sense of calm.

You can practice these techniques together, setting aside dedicated time daily for relaxation exercises. You might also explore guided meditation apps or videos specifically designed for teenagers, which can make the practice more engaging and enjoyable for them.

Besides breathing exercises, encourage your teenager to explore other relaxation techniques that resonate with them. Activities like journaling, drawing, listening to calming music, engaging in hobbies or creative outlets, or spending time in nature can be helpful. By encouraging and participating in these activities with your child, you show them that relaxation and self-care are vital and valuable.

Tip 4: Promote a healthy lifestyle

A healthy lifestyle plays a significant role in managing anxiety. Encourage your teenager to prioritize regular exercise, as physical activity has been shown to reduce anxiety and improve mood.

Find activities they enjoy, whether going for a walk, playing a sport, dancing, or practicing yoga. Physical exercise releases endorphins, which boost mood, help regulate sleep patterns and provide a healthy outlet for stress.

Moreover, a balanced diet is essential for overall well-being, especially mental health. Encourage your teenager to consume nutritious meals that include fruits, vegetables, whole grains, and lean proteins. Limiting the intake of processed foods, sugary snacks, and caffeine can also contribute to a more stable mood and reduce anxiety symptoms.

Tip 5: Encourage social support and connections

Having a supportive social network is crucial for teenagers with anxiety. Encourage your child to maintain friendships and participate in social activities that they enjoy.

Help them identify supportive individuals in their life whom they can confide in and turn to for advice or encouragement. This might include friends, family members, teachers, or mental health professionals.

Consider connecting with support groups or organizations that specialize in anxiety disorders. These groups can give your teenager a sense of community and a platform to share experiences and coping strategies with peers who can relate to their challenges.

Tip 6: Seek professional help when needed

While parental support is essential, it's important to recognize when professional help may be necessary. Consider consulting a mental health professional if your teenager's anxiety significantly impacts their daily life, relationships, or school performance. They can diagnose properly, offer evidence-based treatments, and help your child develop effective coping mechanisms.

A therapist or counselor experienced in working with teenagers can provide valuable support, teaching your child additional strategies to manage anxiety and helping them explore the underlying causes of their anxiety.

Cognitive-behavioral therapy (CBT) is a commonly used therapeutic approach for anxiety and can be particularly effective for teenagers.

In some cases, medication may be prescribed by a psychiatrist to manage severe anxiety symptoms. If this is the case, working closely with a qualified medical professional who can monitor the medication's effectiveness and address any concerns or side effects is crucial.

Remember, every teenager's journey with anxiety is unique, and it may take time to find the right combination of strategies and support that works best for your child.

Stay patient, stay engaged, and most importantly, let your teenager know that you are there to support them every step of the way.

Remember, parents; you can positively shape your teen's mental health journey, so be strong for them.

You can start by prioritizing their well-being, understanding their experiences, and offering unconditional support. Continue to engage in open and non-judgmental conversations with your teenager. Listen attentively to their concerns, fears, and aspirations. Encourage them to embrace their uniqueness and celebrate their achievements, no matter how small. Remind them that setbacks are a natural part of life, and it is through these experiences that they learn and grow.

You can help them develop the resilience needed to navigate the ups and downs of adolescence and emerge as emotionally strong individuals.

Remember to practice self-care as well. By caring for your well-being, you provide a strong foundation for supporting your teenager effectively.

You cannot pour from an empty cup!

You must be attentive to your own mental health needs as well.

Pat yourself on your back for surviving every sleepless night and every breakdown of your child. You deserve it!

CHAPTER 12:

A PARENT'S JOURNEY

"Children have never been very good at listening to their elders, but they have never failed to imitate them."

—James Baldwin

Being a parent is an incredible responsibility, filled with joy and challenges. One of the most challenging aspects can be witnessing your child's struggle with anxiety.

As a parent, your child's anxiety can profoundly impact your well-being and emotional state. It is common to feel anxious and question your parenting techniques, wondering if you are somehow to blame for your child's condition.

This anxiety you experience can then seep into the dynamic of your family, affecting everyone involved.

Research conducted by the National Institute of Health (2014) sheds light on the impact of a child's anxiety on parents.

It reveals that parents' perceptions of family functioning, well-being, and adjustment are significantly affected. Commonly reported consequences include increased worries, depression, fatigue, and health problems.

Relationships may become strained, and personal or social activities may be restricted. The continuous stress of having a child with anxiety can undermine your confidence as a parent, leading to self-blame and feelings of shame.

This, in turn, may limit your participation in social activities or seeking support from others, which are essential sources of strength.

It is essential to recognize that the well-being of parents is closely intertwined with that of their children. This complex interplay involves genetic and environmental factors, such as exposure to stress or trauma.

When parents experience mental health challenges, it often reflects in their interactions with their children.

For instance, parents with depression tend to express more negative emotions towards their children, like anger and irritability. They may also struggle with consistency in discipline and engagement in the parent-child relationship.

Consequently, these stresses at home can contribute to various challenges in children, including depression, anxiety, and behavioral problems.

Parents' psychological well-being is influenced by the stress they experience, including economic difficulties, lack of sufficient childcare, and competing pressures from work and family.

However, social support from family, friends, the community, or the school system can significantly mitigate the negative impact of anxiety and depression on parents' mental health.

The Ripple Effect on Children's Mental Health

We must understand that children whose parents struggle with mental health challenges are more likely to experience anxiety themselves.

The interconnectedness of parent and child mental health is a complex dynamic. When parents receive effective treatment for their own psychiatric conditions, such as cognitive behavioral therapy, it benefits them and positively impacts their children's psychiatric symptoms and overall functioning.

The Power of Inner Work

Parents must first cultivate their consciousness to become the best versions of themselves for their anxious teens.

They must recognize that parenting begins with the adults-the parents-and, not solely with the perceived challenges posed by the "defiant" or "oppositional" child.

They must adopt a thoughtful, mindful mission akin to running a successful organization to lay the foundation for a harmonious parent-child relationship and empower their children to defeat anxiety with resilience.

Understanding Unconscious Parenting

As parents, we must acknowledge that our approach to raising children frequently mirrors our business lives, where strategic planning, self-awareness, and adaptability are paramount.

However, we tend to neglect these principles, often operating on autopilot without considering our actions' profound impact on our children's well-being.

Consciously Embracing Parenthood

To become conscious parents, we must ask ourselves:*What is our parenting mission? How do we manifest this mission in our everyday interactions with our children?*

Just as a successful business leader knows their objective and how to achieve it, parents must also develop a clear vision for their role and strategies.

The Impact of Unconsciousness on Our Children

Unconsciousness in parenting can lead to a heavy toll on our children's emotional well-being. Overindulgence, medication reliance, and labeling are but a few consequences of parental unawareness.

Unresolved needs, unmet expectations, and frustrated dreams inherited from our upbringing can inadvertently shape our children's experiences. Through self-awareness and conscious efforts, we can break the cycle of intergenerational pain and create a wholesome environment for our anxious teens.

The Awakening of Consciousness

Becoming conscious parents necessitates an understanding of our unconscious patterns and conditioning. We may initially resist change, defending our current parenting style.

However, as awareness dawns upon us, we gain the power to redesign the dynamics we share with our children. We recognize that conscious parenting is not about exerting control but cultivating a genuine partnership based on mutual respect and understanding.

Shedding the Illusion of Ego

A fundamental aspect of conscious parenting lies in recognizing and transcending our ego, which often masquerades as our true self. Our ego is our self-image, influenced by others' opinions and conditioning.

We can authentically connect with our children when we distance ourselves from our egos and expectations. This process allows us to tap into our limitless core self, develop genuine connections and dismantle the barriers that separate us from our anxious teens.

Raising Ourselves to Raise Our Children

While it is natural to prioritize raising our children, conscious parenting also requires us to focus on growing ourselves. We must attend to our authentic being, shedding the ego's dominance and control and implementing engaged presence.

Though seemingly less powerful, our children hold the potential to guide us toward our true selves, fueling our personal growth and transformation as parents.

The parent-child relationship becomes a circular journey of mutual enlightenment, where both parties contribute to each other's development.

The Path to Consciousness

Consciousness is not an exclusive gift bestowed upon a fortunate few; rather, it emerges progressively from our unconsciousness through self-reflection and observation. The parent-child relationship presents abundant opportunities for heightened awareness and personal evolution.

We must avail these opportunities to tread the path to consciousness as parents.

Here are some critical practices and principles to guide us on this transformative journey:

Mindful Presence

Cultivate the practice of being fully present with your child. This means setting aside distractions, such as electronic devices, and giving undivided attention to your child when interacting with them. Engage in active listening, showing empathy and understanding, and validating their feelings and experiences. When fully present, you create a safe and nurturing space for your anxious teen to express themselves and feel genuinely seen and heard.

Self-Reflection and Inner Work

Dedicate time to self-reflection and inner work. This involves exploring your past triggers, fears, and unresolved emotions. When you familiarize yourself with your own inner landscape, you can gain clarity on how your experiences may influence your parenting style and the dynamics within your family. Seek support from therapists, counselors, or support groups to assist you in this introspective process.

Emotional Regulation

Cultivate emotional regulation skills for yourself and as a model for your anxious teen. Emotional intelligence involves understanding and managing your own emotions and empathizing with the feelings of others. Through practicing emotional regulation, you can create a calm and stable environment for your child, helping them learn how to monitor their anxiety and emotions.

Authentic Communication

Practice open and authentic communication within your family. Create a space where everyone feels comfortable expressing their thoughts, concerns, and emotions without fear of judgment or punishment. Encourage dialogue and active listening, allowing your anxious teen to share their experiences and perspectives. Be open to learning from your child, as they may offer insights and wisdom that can deepen your understanding and connection.

Setting Healthy Boundaries

Establish clear and healthy boundaries with your anxious teen. Healthy boundaries provide safety and structure while allowing for individual autonomy. Communicate and negotiate boundaries together, considering the needs and preferences of both yourself and your child. Consistency and follow-through are essential in maintaining boundaries, as they provide a sense of predictability and stability for your anxious teen.

Self-Care

Prioritize self-care as an integral part of conscious parenting. Take care of your physical, emotional, and mental well-being, recognizing that your self-care directly impacts your ability to show up as a present and balanced parent. Rear your own interests, engage in activities that bring you joy and relaxation, and seek support when needed. Remember that self-care is not selfish; it is essential for your overall well-being and capacity to support your anxious teen.

Continued Learning and Growth

Commit to ongoing learning and personal growth as a parent. Stay informed about the latest research and resources on anxiety and adolescent development. Attend parenting workshops, read books, and converse with other parents to expand your knowledge and gain new perspectives. Adopt a growth mindset, understanding that parenting is a continuous learning and adaptation journey.

Prioritizing Parents' Well-being

As a parent, it is essential to prioritize your well-being. Just like in the safety instructions on an airplane, where adults are advised to put on their oxygen masks first before assisting others, taking care of your mental health is crucial for promoting your child's well-being.

One concrete action you can take is to seek out family-based treatments. Although it may be challenging, discussing specific referrals for this type of care with your child's pediatrician can be a helpful starting point. If these options are not available, consider seeking individual therapy.

A therapist can provide a safe and supportive space for you to explore your emotions, process guilt or blame, and develop coping strategies to manage the challenges of parenting a child with anxiety.

In addition to professional support, building a strong support network around you is essential. Reach out to family members, friends, or other parents who may be going through similar experiences. Connecting with others who understand and empathize with your situation can provide validation, practical advice, and emotional support.

Lastly, don't hesitate to seek professional help for your child. Anxiety disorders are treatable, and early intervention can make a significant difference. Consult with a mental health professional who specializes in working with children and adolescents to explore appropriate treatment options for your child. This may include therapy, medication, or a combination of both.

Parenting and Adolescents

Navigating the challenging terrain of adolescence can be overwhelming for both parents and teenagers.

Defiant behaviors often emerge during this phase, leaving parents bewildered and unsure how to respond. However, as parents, you must understand that these behaviors stem from unfulfilled needs or underlying fears rather than a purposeful intent to be complicated.

Each child's journey is a unique unfolding of their individuality. Parents should respect and welcome their particular path and empower them to nurture their inner voice while also honoring the voices of others.

In doing so, we equip them with the skills necessary to engage in relationships that reflect a healthy interdependence, laying the foundation for successful intimate relationships in their adult years.

Rejecting the Cookie-Cutter Approach

Parenting is not a one-size-fits-all endeavor. Just as each child possesses a distinct nature, they also require different approaches from their parents. Some may thrive with a soft and gentle approach, while others may need a more assertive style. Letting go of preconceived notions and fantasies about who our children should be allows us to evolve into the parents they need us to be.

Embracing Reality

As parents, we often have expectations and fantasies about who our children will become. However, it is essential to recognize and accept their true nature, even if it deviates from our initial visions. Embracing the reality of our children's unique qualities can be challenging, but it paves the way for a deeper connection and understanding. Adjusting our expectations and recalibrating our approach helps us unapologetically appreciate the individuals our children indeed are.

Acceptance and Behavioral Guidance

Accepting our children's being does not imply passively allowing destructive behaviors. It is the framework upon which we can guide their behavior toward alignment with their essential nature. If a child exhibits defiant behavior out of defiance, firmness may be the appropriate response. However, empathy and understanding become necessary if their behavior stems from struggles with painful emotions. Tailoring our responses to meet their specific needs promotes healthy development.

Acceptance manifests in acknowledging and respecting our children's unique qualities. It may involve accepting their quietness, stubbornness, or need for time to warm up to people.

Whether fearful, rebellious, moody, or gentle, acknowledging and accepting their nature enables us to provide the support they require. When we accept our children's individuality, we create an environment that encourages their personal growth.

Accepting Ourselves

Accepting our children starts with accepting ourselves. Recognizing our limitations, imperfections, and the need for personal growth allows us to become more effective parents. Honoring our being and prioritizing our own joyfulness provides a model for our children to develop their authentic selves. Self-acceptance empowers us to offer genuine acceptance to our children, strengthening the parent-child bond.

The High School Years

As our children transition into high school, the impact of our parenting becomes more apparent. It is during this phase that they assert their personalities with greater intensity. Whether they rebel against strict parenting or seek freedom due to permissiveness, their behavior reflects the unmet needs from earlier years.

Providing a safe space for their individuality and acknowledging our role in their journey becomes indispensable for healing and reconnection.

As I conclude this chapter, I must reflect on the significance of expanding our horizons and engaging in activities beyond ourselves.

Anxiety can be a formidable force, but we can conquer it by shifting our focus outward and embracing a mindset of compassion, service, and exploration.

To the teenagers grappling with anxiety, I implore you to consider the transformative power of volunteering work. Dedicate your time and energy to causes that speak to you personally. This is how you contribute to the betterment of your community and find a sense of purpose and fulfillment that can alleviate the burden of anxiety. Volunteering enables you to connect with others, cultivate empathy, and gain a fresh perspective.

Parents, you play an instrumental role in supporting your anxious teenager's journey toward growth and self-discovery. Encourage and empower them to explore opportunities for community engagement.

Inculcate a spirit of service within your family. You must instill values of kindness and empathy and create a supportive environment that promotes mental well-being. Volunteer together as a family, and witness the positivity it holds for your teenager and yourselves.

Teachers and peers, you can create environments that promote a community mindset. Devise service-learning initiatives where students can actively engage in projects that address social issues.

Inspire discussions on the importance of giving back and create opportunities for students to collaborate on volunteer projects. Create a sense of collective responsibility so you can contribute to your peers' emotional well-being while positively impacting society.

To all of my readers, I urge you to explore self-discovery. Appreciate the beauty of diversity, both within your own community and beyond. Travel, immerse yourself in different cultures, and expand your world understanding.

View the world around you with diverse perspectives to broaden your horizons, challenge preconceived notions, and ultimately alleviate anxiety by tapping into the more extraordinary human experience.

Remember, as you navigate the maze of anxiety, reaching out and extending a helping hand to others can bring about profound healing and growth.

Actively participate in volunteer work, adopt a community mindset, and explore the richness of our planet and its inhabitants so that you may not only find solace and purpose but also contribute to the betterment of our world!

CHAPTER 13:

CONCLUSION

Congratulations on completing your journey through the pages of *"Teen Anxiety: Drop the Rope!"*

Throughout this book, we have indulged in a transformative exploration of anxiety in teenagers, uncovering its underlying causes, recognizing its signs, and equipping both teens and their parents with evidence-based psychotherapy tools to break free from its grip.

We underlined the principles of Cognitive Behavioral Therapy (CBT) and Acceptance and Commitment Therapy (ACT) and empowered ourselves to enrich our lives and overcome the challenges posed by anxiety. Our journey began by acknowledging teen anxiety's pressing problem and its detrimental impact on a young person's life.

As the chapters went on, we delved into the delicate period of adolescence, recognizing its susceptibility to anxiety and the potential long-term consequences if left untreated. We learned to spot the signs and symptoms of anxiety and understand the importance of early intervention and support.

Moving forward, we investigated the various reasons why anxiety manifests in teenagers, encompassing genetic predispositions, environmental factors, trauma, substance abuse, stress, and negative thought patterns.

We unraveled the complex web of anxiety's origins, gained a deeper understanding of its roots, and paved the way for targeted interventions.

With a laser focus on person-centered approaches to treatment, we dived into the benefits and effectiveness of mindfulness, interpersonal psychotherapy, CBT, and ACT.

We appreciated the rewards of mindfulness and discovered the power of present-moment awareness and self-compassion, cultivating resilience and inner peace.

Interpersonal psychotherapy provided valuable insights into the impact of relationships and social interactions on our mental well-being, offering strategies for improving communication and connection.

CBT empowered us to challenge negative thought patterns and develop healthier cognitive habits, while ACT taught us to accept our anxious thoughts and emotions, committing to values-aligned actions and meaningful life.

Recognizing the monumental role of teachers and parents, we explored how schools can support teens with anxiety and how parents can contribute positively to their child's well-being.

We discovered the importance of open communication, empathetic listening, and providing a safe and supportive environment. We learned practical tools and techniques that teachers and parents could employ to assist teens in managing anxiety while also knowing when to seek professional help.

Throughout this journey, we recognized the profound impact that anxiety can have on both teens and their parents. We discussed the emotional toll it takes and emphasized the importance of self-care and seeking support from parents. We appreciated that by tending to our own emotional and mental health, we could better support our children in their journey toward resilience and recovery.

Now, let's discuss why I chose this title for the book.

Do you know what being an anxious teen feels like?

Imagine a scenario where you are engaged in a fierce battle, caught in an intense tug-of-war with a relentless monster. The struggle is exhausting, and fear creeps in as anxiety takes hold of your every thought and emotion.

But what if I told you there's another way? What if you let go and embrace the experience instead of gripping that rope tightly?

By releasing the struggle, you open yourself up to a whole new perspective, a chance to understand the underlying message anxiety has been trying to convey. It's not about denying your emotions or feelings; it's about acknowledging them while shifting your focus to your values, goals, and journey.

With all its challenges and changes, adolescence can be a breeding ground for anxiety. The pressures of school, social dynamics, and personal expectations can sometimes feel overwhelming. It's important to remember that anxiety is not an enemy to be defeated but rather a messenger with valuable insights to offer.

When you drop the rope of struggle, you create space for self-reflection and introspection. You begin to see anxiety as a companion on your journey, urging you to pay attention to aspects of your life that may need nurturing or adjustment. Letting go of the tug-of-war doesn't mean surrendering or giving up.

On the contrary, it's an act of empowerment and self-awareness. It's an invitation to redirect your energy toward what truly matters. Your values, aspirations, and dreams become the focal point, guiding you through the maze of anxiety. It's about finding the strength to listen to your inner voice and trust your intuition.

In the words of the visionary Steve Jobs, who understood the importance of following one's heart,

"The ability to connect the dots and make sense of our journey is often only evident when looking backward, not forward."

This philosophical realization requires trust in the intricacy of life, a belief that the connections will manifest in due course. This trust gives you the courage to defy the noise of others' opinions and prioritize your inner voice.

Sometimes, the path your heart leads you on may diverge from the familiar trails, and that's okay. Take the leap of faith and venture into uncharted territory. As you navigate the complexities of anxiety, remember that your authentic desires and aspirations hold tremendous value. Trust in yourself and prioritize what resonates deep within you. Everything else, no matter how significant it may seem, pales in comparison.

So, dear teens grappling with anxiety and concerned parents, I encourage you to reframe your perspective. See anxiety as an invitation to explore your inner landscape, discover your values, and set meaningful goals. Trust in the process, and you'll find the strength to navigate the tug-of-war with grace and resilience.

Anxiety is undeniably exhausting and can evoke fear. But be vigilant and contemplate what else might be happening beneath the surface. When you release the rope, you open yourself to the possibility of understanding the message that anxiety has been trying to convey.

Letting go of the struggle does not mean denying the existence of emotions and feelings; rather, it means acknowledging them while shifting your focus toward your values, goals, and overall life journey.

Dear teens and parents, the tug-of-war metaphor beautifully captures the essence of anxiety and the power of letting go.

Just imagine holding onto a rope tightly, feeling the strain and resistance as you engage in a relentless battle. Your thoughts, worries, and fears pull you in all directions, leaving you drained and disconnected from what truly matters to you. The tug-of-war exercise demonstrates that fighting against anxiety only perpetuates the struggle. The more you hold on tightly, the more it pulls you away from the things that bring you joy, fulfillment, and growth.

Anxiety has a message for you that can guide you toward self-discovery and personal growth. Letting go of the struggle creates an opportunity to listen to that message. It may be telling you to slow down, set boundaries, or seek support from loved ones. It may be urging you to explore your passions, engage in self-care, or pursue your aspirations.

Trust that the dots of your life will eventually align, even if they may seem scattered and uncertain in the present moment. Allow yourself to trust in your intuition, destiny, or the hidden lessons of life.

Trust the belief that the connections you seek will manifest along your path. This trust empowers you to follow your heart, even if it leads you away from the familiar trials and opinions of others.

Remember, your inner voice holds immense wisdom and understanding of your authentic desires. Amidst the noise of external influences, summon the courage to prioritize what truly speaks to your soul. Trust yourself and cultivate a deep connection with your values, dreams, and aspirations.

Remember that you are not alone on this journey!

Seek support from friends, family, and mental health professionals who can offer guidance and understanding.

As you move forward, I encourage you to practice self-compassion, embrace your strengths, and engage in the therapeutic techniques presented in this book. Use the power of mindfulness, challenge your negative thoughts, accept your emotions, and commit to actions aligned with your values.

Tread the path toward self-discovery and personal growth, knowing that every step forward brings you closer to a life of empowerment, joy, and strength.

May this book serve as a trusted companion for overcoming teen anxiety, and may it empower you to live a life of authenticity, purpose, and well-being.

Remember, you have the strength to drop the rope and reclaim control over your life!

Here are some Teen National Help Hotlines for your consideration:

- https://theyouthalliance.com/resources/help-hotlines/
- https://www.teenline.org/
- https://connectsafely.org/resources-for-youth-in-crisis/
- https://teenlifeline.org/

BIBLIOGRAPHY

1. Ackerman, C. (2017, March 1). ACT: Acceptance and commitment therapy. Positive Psychology. https://positivepsychology.com/act-acceptance-and-commitment-therapy/

2. American Psychological Association. (n.d.). Cognitive-Behavioral Therapy for PTSD. https://www.apa.org/ptsd-guideline/patients-and-families/cognitive-behavioral

3. **Applegate, J. S., & Shapiro, J. R. (2005).** *Neurobiology for clinical social work: Theory and practice*. **WW Norton & Company.**

4. Better Health Channel. (n.d.). Cognitive Behaviour Therapy. https://www.betterhealth.vic.gov.au/health/conditionsandtreatments/cognitive-behaviour-therapy

5. BetterHelp. (2023, March 30). What is acceptance and commitment therapy? https://www.betterhelp.com/advice/therapy/what-is-acceptance-and-commitment-therapy/

6. Biegel, G. M., Brown, K. W., Shapiro, S. L., & Schubert, C. M. (2009). Mindfulness-based stress reduction for the treatment of adolescent psychiatric outpatients: A randomized clinical trial. Journal of consulting and clinical psychology, 77(5), 855–866. https://doi.org/10.1037/a0016241

7. Black, D. S., Slavich, G. M., & Sussman, S. (2015). Mindfulness meditation and the immune system: a systematic review of randomized controlled trials. Annals of the New York Academy of Sciences, 1373(1), 13-24. https://doi.org/10.1111/nyas.12662

8. Bögels, S., & Phares, V. (2008). Fathers' role in the etiology, prevention and treatment of child anxiety: A review and new model. *Clinical psychology review, 28*(4), 539-558.

9. Bowen, S., Witkiewitz, K., Clifasefi, S. L., Grow, J., Chawla, N., Hsu, S. H., ... & Larimer, M. E. (2014). Relative efficacy of mindfulness-based relapse prevention, standard relapse prevention, and treatment as usual for substance use disorders: a randomized clinical trial. JAMA psychiatry, 71(5), 547-556. https://doi.org/10.1001/jamapsychiatry.2014.1

10. Burke, C. A., Langer, E., & Germer, C. S. (2010). Mindfulness-Based Approaches with Children and Adolescents: A Preliminary Review of Current Research in an Emergent Field. Journal of Child and Family Studies, 19(2), 133–144. https://doi.org/10.1007/s10826-009-9282-x

11. Cabral, M. D., & Patel, D. R. (2020). Risk factors and prevention strategies for anxiety disorders in childhood and adolescence. *Anxiety Disorders*, 543-559.

12. Carson, J. W., Carson, K. M., Gil, K. M., & Baucom, D. H. (2004). Mindfulness-based relationship enhancement. Behavior therapy, 35(3), 471-494. https://doi.org/10.1016/S0005-7894(04)80028-0

13. Center for Cognitive Behavioral Therapy. (n.d.). Social anxiety disorder in teenagers. https://cbtpsychology.com/socialanxiety/

14. Chen, X., Li, M., Gong, H., Zhang, Z., & Wang, W. (2021). Factors Influencing Adolescent Anxiety: The Roles of Mothers, Teachers and Peers. International journal of environmental research and public health, 18(24), 13234. https://doi.org/10.3390/ijerph182413234

15. Child Mind Institute. (n.d.). Behavioral Treatment for Kids with Anxiety. https://childmind.org/article/behavioral-treatment-kids-anxiety/

16. Choose Mental Health. (n.d.). Teenager with social anxiety. https://choosementalhealth.org/teenager-with-social-anxiety/

17. Cohen, J. A., Mannarino, A. P., Kinnish, K., & Johnson, J. G. (2017). Effective treatments for PTSD: Practice guidelines from the International Society for Traumatic Stress Studies (2nd ed.). Guilford Press.

18. Cooper, M., McLeod, J., Ogden, G. S., Omylinska-Thurston, J., & Rupani, P. (2015). Client helpfulness interview studies: A guide to exploring client perceptions of change in counselling and psychotherapy. *Unpublished manuscript retrieved from https://www. research gate. net/profile/Mick_Cooper.*

19. Cuijpers, P., Donker, T., Weissman, M. M., Ravitz, P., & Cristea, I. A. (2016). Interpersonal psychotherapy for mental health problems: A comprehensive meta-analysis. The American Journal of Psychiatry, 173(7), 680-687. https://doi.org/10.1176/appi.ajp.2016.15091141

20. Cuijpers, P., Geraedts, A. S., van Oppen, P., Andersson, G., Markowitz, J. C., & van Straten, A. (2013). Interpersonal psychotherapy for depression: A meta-analysis. The American Journal of Psychiatry, 170(6), 581-592. https://doi.org/10.1176/appi.ajp.2012.12081006

21. Cuncic, A. (2020, September 18). Verywell Mind .Social anxiety disorder in children and adolescents. https://www.verywellmind.com/social-anxiety-disorder-in-children-3024430

22. Davidson, R. J., Kabat-Zinn, J., Schumacher, J., Rosenkranz, M., Muller, D., Santorelli, S. F., Urbanowski, F., Harrington, A., Bonus, K., & Sheridan, J. F. (2003). Alterations in brain and immune function produced by mindfulness meditation. Psychosomatic Medicine, 65(4), 564-570. https://doi.org/10.1097/01.PSY.0000077505.67574.E3

23. Dewar, C. (2020, December 14). How does acceptance and commitment therapy help teens struggling with anxiety? Equinox RTC. https://equinoxrtc.com/blog/how-does-acceptance-and-commitment-therapy-help-teens-struggling-with-anxiety/

24. Discovery Mood. (n.d.). Tips for parenting an anxious teen. https://discoverymood.com/blog/tips-parent-anxious-teen/

25. Division 12, Society of Clinical Psychology. (n.d.). Cognitive-Behavioral Therapy for Youth Anxiety: An Overview and Future Directions. https://div12.org/cognitive-behavioral-therapy-for-youth-anxiety-an-overview-and-future-directions/

DOI: 10.1080/02673843.2021.1980067

Ebbert, A. M., Infurna, F. J., & Luthar, S. S. (2019). Mapping developmental changes in perceived parent–adolescent relationship quality throughout middle school and high school. *Development and psychopathology*, *31*(4), 1541-1556.

26. Edsys. (2018, February 28). How teachers can help school students with anxiety. https://www.edsys.in/teachers-help-school-students-with-anxiety/#:~:text=Include%20activities%20that%20ask%20them,to%20help%20them%20stay%20positive.

27. EducationDegree.com. (n.d.). Supporting students with anxiety. https://www.educationdegree.com/articles/supporting-students-with-anxiety/

28. Ehmke, R. (2022, November 3). Child Mind Institute .What is social anxiety? https://childmind.org/article/what-is-social-anxiety/

29. Elliott, R., Bohart, A. C., Watson, J. C., & Greenberg, L. S. (2011). Empathy. Psychotherapy, 48(1), 43-49. https://doi.org/10.1037/a0022187

30. Engle, J. L., & Follette, V. M. (2018). An experimental comparison of two Acceptance and Commitment Therapy (ACT) values exercises to increase values-oriented behavior. Journal of contextual behavioral science, 10, 31-40.

31. Evans, O. (2023, May 11). Simply Psychology. Social anxiety in teens. https://www.simplypsychology.org/social-anxiety-in-teens.html

32. Evolve Treatment Centers. (n.d.). Cognitive Behavioral Therapy (CBT). https://evolvetreatment.com/cognitive-behavioral-therapy/

33. Evolve Treatment Centers. (n.d.). Parent's guide to social anxiety. https://evolvetreatment.com/parent-guides/social-anxiety/

34. Fairburn, C. G., Allen, E., Bailey-Straebler, S., O'Connor, M. E., Cooper, Z., & Bohn, K. (2015). Scaling up psychological treatments: A countrywide test of the online training of therapists. Journal of Medical Internet Research, 17(10), e233. doi: 10.2196/jmir.4066

35. Flannery, S. (2022, December 27). Acceptance and commitment therapy for teens. Child Mind Institute. https://childmind.org/article/acceptance-and-commitment-therapy-for-teens/#:~:text=With%20ACT%2C%20teens%20learn%20to,you%20closer%20to%20your%20goals.

36. Garland, E. L., Farb, N. A., Goldin, P. R., & Fredrickson, B. L. (2015). Mindfulness broadens awareness and builds eudaimonic meaning: A process model of mindful positive emotion regulation. Psychological Inquiry, 26(4), 293-314. https://doi.org/10.1080/1047840X.2015.1064294

37. Glasofer, D. (2021, September 21). Acceptance and commitment therapy for generalized anxiety disorder. Verywell

Mind. https://www.verywellmind.com/acceptance-commitment-therapy-gad-1393175

38. Goldberg, S. B., Tucker, R. P., Greene, P. A., Davidson, R. J., Kearney, D. J., & Simpson, T. L. (2018). Mindfulness-based cognitive therapy for the treatment of current depressive symptoms: A meta-analysis. Cognitive Behaviour Therapy, 47(3), 178-193. https://doi.org/10.1080/16506073.2017.1409082

39. Good Therapy. (2018, February 12). Acceptance and commitment therapy (ACT). https://www.goodtherapy.org/learn-about-therapy/types/acceptance-commitment-therapy

40. Halliburton, A. E., & Cooper, L. D. (2015). Applications and adaptations of Acceptance and Commitment Therapy (ACT) for adolescents. Journal of Contextual Behavioral Science, 4(1), 1-11.

41. Han, T. (2021, June). Analysis of Teen Anxiety with Regard to COVID-19 Pandemic. In *2021 2nd International Conference on Mental Health and Humanities Education (ICMHHE 2021)* (pp. 256-261). Atlantis Press.

42. Harnett, P. H., Reid, S. C., Loxton, N. J., & Lee, N. (2016). The efficacy of Acceptance and Commitment Therapy for at-risk adolescents: A randomized controlled trial. Journal of Contextual Behavioral Science, 5(2), 111-121. https://doi.org/10.1016/j.jcbs.2016.02.003

43. Harris, R. (n.d.). Acceptance and commitment therapy (ACT). https://www.psychotherapy.net/article/Acceptance-and-Commitment-Therapy-ACT

44. Healthline. (n.d.). Cognitive Behavioral Therapy (CBT). https://www.healthline.com/health/cognitive-behavioral-therapy#things-to-keep-in-mind

45. Herd, T and Font, S. (2022, December 1). How parents can play a key role in the prevention and treatment of teen mental health problems. The Conversation. https://theconversation.com/how-parents-can-play-a-key-role-in-the-prevention-and-treatment-of-teen-mental-health-problems-192927

46. Hofmann, S. G., & Smits, J. A. (2017). Cognitive-behavioral therapy for adult anxiety disorders: A meta-analysis of randomized placebo-controlled trials. The Journal of Clinical Psychiatry, 78(8), e760-e766. https://doi.org/10.4088/JCP.16r10783

47. Hölzel, B. K., Carmody, J., Vangel, M., Congleton, C., Yerramsetti, S. M., Gard, T., & Lazar, S. W. (2011). Mindfulness practice leads to increases in regional brain gray matter density. Psychiatry research: Neuroimaging, 191(1), 36-43. https://doi.org/10.1016/j.pscychresns.2010.08.006

48. https://www.crossway.org/articles/a-parents-role-in-teen-anxiety/

49. Johnson, L. E., & Greenberg, M. T. (2013). Parenting and Early Adolescent Internalizing: The Importance of Teasing Apart Anxiety and Depressive Symptoms. The Journal of early adolescence, 33(2), 201–226. https://doi.org/10.1177/0272431611435261

50. Kaplan, A., Reynolds, S., & Caviglia, G. (2015). Interpersonal psychotherapy for social anxiety disorder: An open pilot study. Journal of Contemporary Psychotherapy, 45(4), 203-210. doi: 10.1007/s10879-015-9301-x

51. Kendall, P. C., & Peterman, J. S. (2015). CBT for adolescents with anxiety: Mature yet still developing. *American Journal of Psychiatry, 172*(6), 519-530.

52. Kensit, D. A. (2000). Rogerian theory: A critique of the effectiveness of pure client-centred therapy. *Counselling Psychology Quarterly, 13*(4), 345-351.

53. Keohan, E. (2021, December, 21). Talkspace. Social anxiety in teens: Causes, signs, and treatment options. https://www.talkspace.com/blog/social-anxiety-in-teens/

54. Khoury, B., Lecomte, T., Fortin, G., Masse, M., Therien, P., Bouchard, V., Chapleau, M. A., Paquin, K., & Hofmann, S. G. (2013). Mindfulness-based therapy: A comprehensive meta-analysis. Clinical Psychology Review, 33(6), 763–771. https://doi.org/10.1016/j.cpr.2013.05.005

55. KidsHealth. (2022, February). Social phobia (social anxiety disorder) in teens. https://kidshealth.org/en/teens/social-phobia.html

56. Lazary, J., Eszlari, N., Juhasz, G., & Bagdy, G. (2019). A functional variant of CB2 receptor gene interacts with childhood trauma and the FAAH gene on anxious and depressive phenotypes. *Journal of Affective Disorders, 257*, 716-722.

57. Levitt, H. M., Butler, M., Hill, T., & Hausmann, A. (2006). Effects of person-centered and experiential therapies on the reduction of depressive and anxiety symptoms in high school students: A randomized controlled trial. Journal of Counseling Psychology, 53(2), 209-218. https://doi.org/10.1037/0022-0167.53.2.209

58. Lipschitz, J. M., Markowitz, J. C., Cherry, S., Foa, E. B., & Mannarino, A. (2019). Treatment of childhood comorbidity in a randomized controlled trial of interpersonal psychotherapy for depressed adolescents. Journal of the American Academy of Child & Adolescent Psychiatry, 58(3), 283-293. https://doi.org/10.1016/j.jaac.2018.10.014

59. Markowitz, J. C., Petkova, E., Neria, Y., Van Meter, P. E., Zhao, Y., Hembree, E., ... & Marshall, R. D. (2015). Is exposure necessary? A randomized clinical trial of interpersonal psychotherapy for PTSD. American Journal of Psychiatry, 172(5), 430-440. doi: 10.1176/appi.ajp.2014.14070818

60. Martin, L., Viljoen, M., Kidd, M., & Seedat, S. (2014). Are childhood trauma exposures predictive of anxiety sensitivity in school attending youth?. *Journal of Affective Disorders, 168*, 5-12.

61. Matthewson, M., Smith, R., & Montgomery, I. (2012). Does the Parent–Child Relationship Contribute to Children's and Parents' Anxiety? *Journal of Relationships Research, 3*, 1-9. doi:10.1017/jrr.2012.2

62. McLeod, B. D., & Jensen-Doss, A. (2015). The efficacy of psychosocial treatments for children and adolescents with anxiety disorders: A systematic review and meta-analysis. Behavior Therapy, 46(3), 295-312. https://doi.org/10.1016/j.beth.2014.12.009

63. McLeod, S. (2015). Person centered therapy. *Simply Psychology*. Retrieved from https://www.simplypsychology.org/client-centred-therapy.html Person-centered therapy

64. Medical News Today. School anxiety: Causes, symptoms, and treatments. https://www.medicalnewstoday.com/articles/school-anxiety#seeking-help

65. Mental Health Center for Kids. (n.d.). School anxiety in teenagers. https://mentalhealthcenterkids.com/blogs/articles/school-anxiety-in-teenagers/

66. Middle Earth. (2021, May 10). A parent's guide to teen anxiety. Retrieved from https://middleearthnj.org/2021/05/10/a-parents-guide-to-teen-anxiety/

67. Mufson, L., Dorta, K. P., Wickramaratne, P., Nomura, Y., Olfson, M., & Weissman, M. M. (2010). A randomized

effectiveness trial of interpersonal psychotherapy for depressed adolescents. Archives of General Psychiatry, 67(12), 1250-1260. https://doi.org/10.1001/archgenpsychiatry.2010.168

68. Murray, D. (2020, October 30). A parent's role in teen anxiety. Crossway.

69. Nash, J. (n.d.). Positive Psychology. Clean and Dirty Discomfort Diary https://positive.b-cdn.net/wp-content/uploads/2022/01/The-Clean-and-Dirty-Discomfort-Diary.pdf

70. Nash, J., & Lancia, G. (2022, January 14). ACT Therapy Techniques: 14+ Interventions for Your Sessions. Positive Psychology. https://positivepsychology.com/act-techniques/

71. Newport Academy. (2020, July 22). ACT for teens: Acceptance and commitment therapy. https://www.newportacademy.com/resources/mental-health/act-for-teens/

72. Newport Academy. (n.d.). Back to school anxiety. https://www.newportacademy.com/resources/mental-health/back-to-school-anxiety/

73. Noel, S. (2018). Person-centered therapy (Rogerian therapy). *Retrieved March, 11*, 2019.

74. Pascoe, M. C., Thompson, D. R., & Jenkins, Z. M. (2017). Mindfulness mediates the physiological markers of stress: Systematic review and meta-analysis. Journal of Psychiatric Research, 95, 156-178. https://doi.org/10.1016/j.jpsychires.2017.08.004

75. Pegg, S., Hill, K., Argiros, A., Olatunji, B. O., & Kujawa, A. (2022). Cognitive Behavioral Therapy for Anxiety Disorders in Youth: Efficacy, Moderators, and New Advances in Predicting Outcomes. *Current Psychiatry Reports*, 1-7.

76. Perry, B. D. (2009). Examining child maltreatment through a neurodevelopmental lens: Clinical applications of the neurosequential model of therapeutics. *Journal of Loss and Trauma, 14*(4), 240-255.

77. Polaris Teen Center. (2019, February 27). Social anxiety in teens. https://polaristeen.com/articles/social-anxiety-in-teens/

78. Positive Psychology. (n.d.). CBT: Cognitive Behavioral Therapy Techniques & Worksheets. https://positivepsychology.com/cbt-cognitive-behavioral-therapy-techniques-worksheets/

79. PositivePsychology.com. (2020). Personal Values Worksheet [PDF]. https://positivepsychology.com/wp-content/uploads/2020/11/Personal-Values-Worksheet.pdf

80. Psych Central. (n.d.). In-Depth: Cognitive-Behavioral Therapy. https://psychcentral.com/lib/in-depth-cognitive-behavioral-therapy#is-it-right-for-me

81. Psychology Today. (n.d.). Acceptance and commitment therapy (ACT). March 21, 2022, https://www.psychologytoday.com/intl/therapy-types/acceptance-and-commitment-therapy

82. Psychology Today. (n.d.). Cognitive-Behavioral Therapy (CBT). https://www.psychologytoday.com/intl/basics/cognitive-behavioral-therapy

83. Psychology Tools. (n.d.). What Is CBT? https://www.psychologytools.com/self-help/what-is-cbt/

84. Purcell, A. (2021, June 28). ACT Metaphors: A Guide to Acceptance and Commitment Therapy. Mental Health @ Home. https://mentalhealthathome.org/2021/06/28/act-metaphors/

85. Putwain, D. W. (2007). Test anxiety in UK schoolchildren: Prevalence and demographic patterns. *British Journal of Educational Psychology, 77*(3), 579-593.

86. Rogers, C. (1959). A theory of therapy, personality and interpersonal relationships as developed in the client-centered framework. In (ed.) S. Koch, *Psychology: A study of a science. Vol. 3: Formulations of the person and the social context.* New York: McGraw Hill.

87. Schluger, A (n.d.). Anxiety in children and teens. HelpGuide. org. https://www.helpguide.org/articles/anxiety/anxiety-in-children-and-teens.htm#:~:text=Research%20conducted%20in%202021%20highlighted,ease%20their%20stress%20and%20anxiety.

88. Scott, E. (2022, April 22).

89. Segal, Z. V., Williams, J. M., & Teasdale, J. D. (2010). Mindfulness-based cognitive therapy for depression: a new approach to preventing relapse. Guilford Press. DOI: 10.1093/med:psych/9780199665564.001.0001

90. Seligman, L. D., & Ollendick, T. H. (2011). Cognitive-behavioral therapy for anxiety disorders in youth. *Child and adolescent psychiatric clinics of North America, 20*(2), 217–238. https://doi.org/10.1016/j.chc.2011.01.003

91. Semple, R. J., Lee, J., Rosa, D., & Miller, L. F. (2010). A randomized trial of mindfulness-based cognitive therapy for children: promoting mindful attention to enhance social-emotional resiliency in children. Journal of Child and Family Studies, 19(2), 218-229. https://doi.org/10.1007/s10826-009-9301-y

92. Shafir, H. (2023, April 5). Acceptance and commitment therapy. Retrieved September 10, 2021, from https://www.choosingtherapy.com/acceptance-and-

commitment-therapy/#:~:text=Acceptance%20and%20Commitment%20Therapy%20was,Hayes%20called%20Relational%20Frame%20Theory.

93. Simply Psychology. (n.d.). Cognitive Therapy. https://www.simplypsychology.org/cognitive-therapy.html

94. Starleaf, J. (2021, August 23). National Social Anxiety Center. Social anxiety in teenagers: How to recognize it and find appropriate support. https://nationalsocialanxietycenter.com/2021/08/23/social-anxiety-in-teenagers-how-to-recognize-it-and-find-appropriate-support/

95. Stoddard, J. A., & Afari, N. (2014). The Big Book of ACT Metaphors: a practitioner's guide to experiential exercises and metaphors in Acceptance and Commitment Therapy. New Harbinger Publications.

96. Swaim, E. (2022, September 19). Acceptance and commitment therapy (ACT). Healthline. https://www.healthline.com/health/mental-health/acceptance-and-commitment-therapy#how-to-try-it

97. Swain, J., Hancock, K., Dixon, A., & Bowman, J. (2015). Acceptance and Commitment Therapy for children: A systematic review of intervention studies. Journal of Contextual Behavioral Science, 4(2), 73-85.

98. Swain, J., Hancock, K., Dixon, A., Koo, S., & Bowman, J. (2013). Acceptance and commitment therapy for anxious children and adolescents: Study protocol for a randomized controlled trial. Trials, 14(1), 1-12.

99. Tang, Y. Y., Hölzel, B. K., & Posner, M. I. (2015). The neuroscience of mindfulness meditation. Nature Reviews Neuroscience, 16(4), 213-225. https://doi.org/10.1038/nrn3916

100. Teach.com. (2022, April 25). Helping students with anxiety disorders. https://teach.com/resources/helping-students-with-anxiety-disorders/

101. The School of Life. (n.d.). Nietzsche, regret and amor fati. https://www.theschooloflife.com/article/nietzsche-regret-and-amor-fati/#:~

102. Towe-Goodman, N. R., Franz, L., Copeland, W., Angold, A., & Egger, H. (2014). Perceived family impact of preschool anxiety disorders. Journal of the American Academy of Child and Adolescent Psychiatry, 53(4), 437–446. https://doi.org/10.1016/j.jaac.2013.12.017

103. Tsabary, S. (2010). The Conscious Parent: Transforming Ourselves, Empowering Our Children. Namaste Publishing.

104. Twenge, J. M. (2019). More time on technology, less happiness? Associations between digital-media use and psychological well-being. *Current Directions in Psychological Science*, *28*(4), 372-379.

105. Vallejo, M. (2022, December 20)

106. Vaughan-Smith, H. (n.d.). They Are the Future . Social anxiety in teenagers. https://www.theyarethefuture.co.uk/social-anxiety-in-teenager/

107. Verywell Family. (2022, September 21). Social causes of school anxiety. https://www.verywellfamily.com/social-causes-of-school-anxiety-3145171

108. Verywell Mind. (n.d.). Therapy for Teens: How It Works, Types, and More. https://www.verywellmind.com/therapy-for-teens-2610410

109. Verywell Mind. (n.d.). What Is Cognitive-Behavior Therapy (CBT)? https://www.verywellmind.com/what-is-cognitive-behavior-therapy-2795747

110. Weare, K., & Nind, M. (2011). Mental health promotion and problem prevention in schools: what does the evidence say? Health Promotion International, 26(Suppl 1), i29-i69. https://doi.org/10.1093/heapro/dar075

111. WebMD. (2021, April 9). What is acceptance and commitment therapy? https://www.webmd.com/mental-health/what-is-acceptance-and-commitment-therapy

112. White, T. R. (2013). Digital social media detox (DSMD): Responding to a culture of interconnectivity. In *Social media and the new academic environment: Pedagogical challenges* (pp. 414-430). IGI Global.

113. Wilfley, D. E., Welch, R. R., Stein, R. I., Spurrell, E. B., Cohen, L. R., Saelens, B. E., ... & Matt, G. E. (2002). A randomized comparison of group cognitive-behavioral therapy and group interpersonal psychotherapy for the treatment of overweight individuals with binge-eating disorder. Archives of General Psychiatry, 59(8), 713-721. https://doi.org/10.1001/archpsyc.59.8.713

114. Yaffe, Y. (2021). A narrative review of the relationship between parenting and anxiety disorders in children and adolescents. *International Journal of Adolescence and Youth*, *26*(1), 449-459.

115. Young, J. F., Benas, J. S., Schueler, C. M., Gallop, R., Gillham, J. E., & Mufson, L. (2016). A randomized depression prevention trial comparing interpersonal psychotherapy—adolescent skills training to group counseling in schools. Journal of the American Academy of Child & Adolescent Psychiatry, 55(7), 603-611. https://doi.org/10.1016/j.jaac.2016.04.012

116. Zeidan, F., Johnson, S. K., Diamond, B. J., David, Z., & Goolkasian, P. (2010). Mindfulness meditation improves cognition: Evidence of brief mental training. Consciousness and cognition, 19(2), 597-605. https://doi.org/10.1016/j.concog.2010.03.014